Hospice
Complete Care for the
Terminally Ill

Hospice

Complete Care for the Terminally Ill

Jack McKay Zimmerman, M.D., F.A.C.S.
Church Hospital, Baltimore

Contributions by
Paul S. Dawson, M.S.
Kathleen Anne Roche, R.N., M.A.
Gloria R. Cameron, M.H.A.

Foreword by
Dame Cicely Saunders

Urban & Schwarzenberg
Baltimore-Munich   1981

Urban & Schwarzenberg, Inc.
7 E. Redwood Street
Baltimore, Maryland 21202
USA

Urban & Schwarzenberg
Pettenkoferstrasse 18
D-8000 München 2
Germany

R
726.8
.Z55

Printed in the United States of America

Library of Congress Cataloging in Publication Data

Zimmerman, Jack McKay.
    Hospice: complete care for the terminally ill.

    Includes index.
    1. Terminal care.   2. Terminal care facilities.
    I. Title. [DNLM: 1. Hospices. 2. Terminal care.
    WX 28.61 Z72h]
    R726.8.Z55   616′.029   81-1375
    ISBN 0-8067-2211-8   AACR2

ISBN 0-8067-2211-8 (Baltimore)

ISBN 3-541-72211-8 (Munich)

This book is dedicated to
DORIS
Co-author of all that is best in my life

Contents

Foreword

The present day hospice is a program rather than a place, an attitude expressed in a growing expertise that is being established in many different ways. It has developed out of the work of homes or hospices founded on both sides of the Atlantic at the turn of the century for patients with terminal cancer and tuberculosis. As the hospitals became more involved with acute care and turned these patients away to Poor Law or equivalent institutions, these turn-of-the-century hospices grew up.

Hospice therapeutics may be traced back to the classic *The Care of the Aged, the Dying and the Dead* written by a family doctor for students of Harvard Medical School (Worcester, 1935), but apart from a few articles from the homes and a Harveian Oration (Gavey, 1952) little was written before 1960, when work developed at St. Joseph's Hospice began to be published (Saunders, 1960). By this time advances in the treatment of malignant disease had offered longer-term control, better palliation and sometimes cure to many patients, while for others it had greatly lengthened the time of ill health and dependence and led to mental as well as physical suffering. The trend for death to occur in the hospital rather than in the patient's own home isolated him from all that was familiar, often without the understanding or treatment appropriate to his special needs (Hinton, 1963). The fear of a painful and isolated death was widespread.

The work in pain control that was observed at St. Luke's Hospital (an early hospice) from 1948 onwards was developed in St. Joseph's Hospice (founded in 1905) after 1958. By then it was possible to exploit the therapeutic advances of the 1950's: new psychotropic drugs, cancer chemotherapy, palliative radiotherapy, the techniques of the new Pain Clinics, and a greater knowledge of family responses to stress and bereavement in a new approach to the terminally ill. St. Christopher's opened in 1967 as the first research and teaching hospice. From the first it focused on the family as the unit of care and, where possible, as part of the caring team, as well as upon the nature of terminal pain, its better understanding and therefore more effective treatment. Alongside this came a revival of the concept of the ''good death,'' attention to the achievements that a patient could still make in the face of his physical deterioration, and awareness of the spiritual dimension of his final search for meaning. Since then the work has spread in a wide variety of interpretations and has grown into the Hospice Movement.

⌐A modern hospice, whether it is a separate unit or ward, a home care or hospital team, aims to enable a patient to live to the limit of his potential in physical strength, mental and emotional capacity and social relationships. It offers an alternative form of treatment to the acute care of a general hospital, not in opposition but as a further resource for those for whom the usual acute hospital care is no longer appropriate. It is the alternative to the negative and socially dangerous suggestion that a patient with an incurable disease likely to cause suffering should have the legal option of actively hastened death or euthanasia⌐

For the present it appears that a limited number of research and teaching hospices will be needed to establish recognized techniques and standards of care that can be interpreted in the home as well as in other settings. A hospice aim from the start has been that such work should become part of general medical and nursing teaching and this book is an important step in that direction. Perhaps the team or unit that is part of a hospital complex such as is here described has the greatest opportunity to integrate with and enrich general practice. The knowledge it contains will form a valuable reference to those working elsewhere in the field.

So far the American hospice has limited itself almost entirely to the dying cancer patient and his family. St. Christopher's, like St. Joseph's, has always had a mixed community of patients. Let us hope that the attitude of skilled attention and respect enshrined in this book will spread to include all those for whom the resources of acute medicines have become irrelevant, but who need help to complete their lives with a sense of personal worth to the end (Vanderpool, 1978).

Spring 1981

DAME CICELY SAUNDERS

References

Gavey, C.J.: *The Management of the "Hopeless" Case*. Lewis, London (1952)

Hinton, J.M.: The Physical and Mental Distress of the Dying. Quart J Med NS Vol. 32, 1 (1963)

Saunders, C.: *Care of the Dying*. Nursing Times Reprint, Macmillan, London (1960)

Vanderpool, H.Y.: The Ethics of Terminal Care. JAMA, Vol. 239, 850–852 (1978)

Worcester, A.: *The Care of the Aged, the Dying, and the Dead*. Thomas, Springfield (1935); Blackwells, London (1961)

Acknowledgments

The preparation of this book has required the help of many people in many ways.

To Dame Cicely Saunders, I shall always be deeply indebted, not just for her unique contribution to this field, but for her personal instruction and encouragement. From Dr. Thomas West, I have learned much about how hospice care really works. The entire staff at St. Christopher's has, with good spirit, always been ready to help and give advice.

Dr. Eric Wilkes' delightful clarity of expression, graciousness and imaginative approach have placed the stamp of St. Luke's in Sheffield upon the Church Hospice program in Baltimore. My first visit to a hospice was to one which shuns the term; at St. Barnabas Home I had from Dr. F.R. Gusterson a superb and colorful introduction to hospice care. Dr. Richard Lamerton's incisive style often expresses what others are thinking but can't quite say. Dr. Balfour Mount's visit to Church Hospital several years ago was a turning point for our entire program and for myself personally; he made it all seem possible and showed us a model which was applicable to our situation.

Hospice care exists at Church Hospital because Reverend Paul Dawson had both the vision and the perseverance to make it a reality. With her organizational skill Gloria Cameron made it possible to convert an idea into a functioning program. The third contributing author, Kathleen Roche, has brought to Church Hospital two valuable ingredients of our program: expertise in both home care and thanatology.

The late Helen Fowler was an inspiration to us all. She was part of Paul Dawson's original team and at the beginning was a one-woman home care program. Her devotion to her patients and her own valiant battle against cancer were a model of life as it should be lived.

From the start, Dr. Bernard Yukna has been our hospice physician. He has brought to this work an understanding compassion which has been critical to the success of the program. He has quickly become one of the most knowledgeable people in the world about symptom relief in the terminally ill. Bonnie Ray, our clinical nurse practitioner, not only makes the program operate from day to day but makes it do so vigorously and harmoniously. Maureen and George Mason were both instrumental in the founding of Church Hospital's hospice program. George, as Vice President of the hospital when the hospice program was conceived, guided its early steps. Maureen's tireless work as a volunteer and as an articulate spokeswoman for the program have been invaluable. Miriam Wallace, our social worker, has always had the interests of the patient and the program uppermost in her mind. Each of the other members of the hospice team, including the professional and volunteer staff on Barton 5 and the Home Health Staff, has been a key part of this book; they do the work I write about.

Fred Wehr, Director of Development and Public Relations, has been our interface with much of the community and with the media; in addition he has provided valuable questions and advice. Father Joseph Krach, our Catholic chaplain, has played a critical role in the program from its inception. Mrs. Zu McBee, director of volunteers, has been instrumental in the function of our program. Mrs. Joyce O'Shea, director of nursing, has provided leadership in meeting the nursing needs of the program and thoughtful help to the author in reviewing portions of the manuscript. Lady Mary Ward has not only been a friend to the Church Hospital program but has stimulated us and given encouragement. Dr. Josephina Magno's leadership in hospice work nationally and her kind assistance locally have meant a great deal.

Without the enthusiasm and prodding of my medical school classmate and friend, Dr. A. Jefferson Penfield, this book would not have been written.

There also would have been no book without the patience and indulgence of my secretaries. Carol Tracey gathered, reviewed and organized material. Ruth Ann Rochlitz typed tirelessly for an author who was an unfortunate combination of compulsive and disorganized.

A very special expression of thanks must of course go to our patients and their families. They have been the central characters in all of this and it is from them that we have learned the most.

Preface

This book is designed to be of assistance to those who are, in one way or another, concerned with the care of the terminally ill patient. Most particularly, it is directed at those who would like to know more about how the hospice concept may contribute to the comfort of the dying patient and his family.

Its primary purpose is to serve as a guide for all who are interested in, who are developing or who are involved in the early stages of a hospice program. However, we hope that even those who have had some experience in hospice care may find something of value.

Although written from a physician's viewpoint, this volume is intended to be useful to all who are involved in the care of the dying patient. This deserves particular emphasis because hospice care is, by its nature, multidisciplinary; it requires the active participation of nursing personnel, social workers, volunteers, administrators, trustees and others. I have tried to take an orderly and logical approach in presentation of material, but some sections will be of more interest and value to certain readers than will others.

Although some effort has been directed at providing a comprehensive picture of hospice care for the terminally ill, my main thrust has been toward practical considerations in dealing successfully with the dying patient. In order to do this I have begun by identifying current problems in the management of the terminally ill and providing a brief overview of the way in which hospice care tries to respond to these problems. A description of our experience in the Church Hospital Hospice Care Program provides a picture of one hospice. Consideration is then directed at the principles and practices of hospice care, including symptom control and meeting the emotional and psychosocial needs of the patient and his family. The composition of the hospice care team is reviewed, as are the cardinal features of inpatient and outpatient care. Attention is then directed at the organization, financing and staffing of a hospice care program. The book concludes with an attempt to answer some of the commonly asked questions about hospice care today and a brief look at future developments in the care of the terminally ill.

This may seem ambitious, but it is undertaken in the belief that we have reached a point in the care of the dying patient where such an analysis is valuable. No effort is made here to give a detailed chronological history of hospice care, nor to make comparison between various types of hospices. This book is simply founded on the premise that our experience speaks to some of the issues in the care of the dying and that the results of that experience may be of help to those who have some interest in or responsibility for treatment of patients terminally ill from malignancy.

The reader will quickly perceive that my contributors and I have written from the perspective of a hospice care program which is hospital based and which, for sound and practical reasons, has confined its initial commitment to patients terminally ill with malignancy. Those of us who have been involved with the Church Hospital hospice program believe in the value of hospital-based programs, while conceding that under some circumstances other models are appropriate. There are both advantages and disadvantages to restricting a developing program to the treatment of advanced malignancy.

For the most part, the approach I have taken is to provide basic information on the current status of hospice care. However, with respect to some of the controversies and uncertainties about hospice care, I have deliberately been provocative. It is often in response to this approach that the reader gains the clearest insights.

The approach here has been to be thorough in the sense of touching upon the important and practical matters in care of the terminally ill. However, in the interests of being helpful, I have tried to be concise. Therefore the coverage is not exhaustive. Many of the topics dealt with here deserve deeper consideration than would be appropriate in a book such as this. Some are legitimately the topics of books themselves.

The effort here is to provide only a framework upon which one may build. The current state of knowledge about the care of the terminally ill and the diversity of experience in hospice care thus far do not permit us to do more at present. Furthermore, there will always be the need to adapt to local circumstances. I have tried to provide a sound framework based upon a careful look at our own experience and that of others.

Let there be no misunderstanding. Commitment to improved care for patients terminally ill from malignant disease in no way de-emphasizes the importance of efforts directed toward the prevention, early detection and curative treatment of cancer, nor toward the rehabilitation of patients undergoing curative treatment. A major thesis of this book is, in fact, the need for co-ordination, co-operation and cross-fertilization between curative and palliative care.

There clearly is much about hospice which is international and catholic. However, certain things such as drug names, health care delivery organization and financing, etc., are peculiarly national. In these respects this book has been written with an American audience in mind.

The reader has a right to know something about the vantage point from which the author views his subject, as this is often helpful information in evaluating the text. I am a general and thoracic surgeon who has been Chief of Surgery at

Church Hospital for more than 15 years. I am Associate Professor of Surgery at Johns Hopkins University and Surgeon at the Johns Hopkins Hospital. My primary commitments are to the practice of surgery, to teaching and to the administration of my service. As a surgeon I have had a long-standing interest in the role of surgery in the palliation of malignancy, most particularly as it concerns carcinoma of the esophagus, lung and pancreas. I also serve as chairman of the Church Hospital Hospice Care Committee and have, from the inception of our hospice program, been the attending physician for a portion of our hospice patients. I have thus viewed Church Hospital's hospice program both as a participating staff member and as an observer. Recognizing that it is presumptuous and hazardous for a relative newcomer—and a part-time one at that—to write about hospice care, I was reinforced in my resolve to undertake this venture by the generous provision of assistance from every member of our hospice care team, each of whom gave unselfishly of his knowledge and experience to make this book possible.

Those of us involved in hospice care today stand on the shoulders of the pioneer workers in England, Canada and the United States. Our debt to them is immense. There is still much for this and future generations to learn about the care of the terminally ill. We hope that in the future, others will be standing on our shoulders.

Spring 1981

JACK MCKAY ZIMMERMAN

1. Problems in the Care of the Dying Patient— Hospice Care as a Response

Problems in the Care of the Patient Dying from Cancer

In recent years, research scientists and clinicians alike have devoted much attention to the prevention, early detection and curative treatment of malignant disease. These efforts have met with varying success. There are many patients who at the time they initially come to a physician's attention or subsequent to efforts at curative treatment are incurable. The palliative care of such patients is the subject of this book.

Malignant disease beyond the possibility of cure is not uncommon. Patients in this situation are part of the common experience not only of medical personnel but of most people. There are few of us whose lives have not been touched by someone dying of cancer. Looked at from a statistical standpoint, cancer ranks second to diseases of the heart among the leading causes of death in the United States. The average death rate from cancer per 100,000 population per year is about 180, which means there will be an estimated 400,000 deaths from cancer in the United States in 1980. Put differently, malignant disease accounts for about 20% of all deaths. Death from cancer occurs in all age groups; of the 7645 such deaths in Maryland in 1978, 43% were individuals under 65 years of age.

It is also part of our common experience that care for terminally ill patients is fraught with difficulties and often is less than ideal. There is clearly room for improvement.

There are a number of reasons, both philosophical and practical, that palliative care of patients with advanced malignancy is less than optimal. The reasons for and the nature of suboptimal care for the dying patient have been well described by a number of authors, including Mount (1976a) and Ryder and Ross (1977). Graphic and touching reports based on personal experience have been provided in books such as John Gunther's *Death Be Not Proud* (1949) and Stewart Alsop's *Stay of Execution* (1973). Because the reader has doubtless already recognized

1

these problems and perceived the need for improvement, we will not deal with this matter exhaustively, but will only make a few observations.

The human situation of terminal illness must be looked at in a number of different dimensions. Terminal illness has both medical and non-medical aspects. The disease process, its symptoms and its ramifications are clearly medical matters. The impact of both the illness and impending death on the family structure and family finances are not, strictly speaking, medical matters. Furthermore, some of the problems which occur in the terminally ill are related to impending death (one's attitude toward death and one's practical and emotional preparation for it), but the illness itself, entirely aside from the fact that it will be lethal, has an impact upon the dying patient and his family. Pre-existing problems anteceding the terminal illness, although not immediately related to illness or death, are thrown into sharper focus and sometimes require more definitive resolution because of the terminal illness. Finally, dying must be looked at as involving *both the patient and his family*. Both are clearly involved in the dying process and the long range effect of the patient's death on the family may be considerable.

When each of the dimensions of terminal illness is examined separately, the origin and nature of the problems relating to it become clearer and perhaps a bit easier to comprehend, if not to accept.

Looked at from a medical standpoint, terminal illness from cancer is clearly the result of a serious and advanced disease. The immense technological improvements of recent years have developed the capacity for cure of many previously disabling or lethal conditions; it is only natural that our system of health care delivery has responded by organizing itself to facilitate such cure. This is not only natural, but fortunate and commendable. There has, however, been an unfortunate by-product; the provision of supportive palliative care for the terminally ill has suffered. It has suffered in a number of ways. As medical care has become increasingly technologically sophisticated, the most advanced care has become institutionally based. As a consequence, there is a tendency to place all severely ill patients in the hospital rather than at home. Hospitals tend to be threatening, restrictive and impersonal. Furthermore, in the hospital setting the availability of a vast panorama of medications and other therapeutic techniques can make it difficult to withhold treatment measures. Also, the inroads which curative techniques are making against malignant disease sometimes makes it difficult for physicians to determine definitely whether or not the patient has passed beyond the point of cure. Increasing specialization, itself a by-product of expanding technology, has led to less continuity of care. In subtle but definite ways, probably only in part related to technological advance, the interpersonal relationships between those providing care and patients have deteriorated. This development hampers relief of symptoms, which depends upon communication between patient and care provider. Furthermore, in recent decades clinical scientists have directed less attention to symptom relief than to disease control. All of these factors have combined to impede the provision of optimal palliative care to patients beyond the hope of cure.

When one looks at the non-medical aspects of the care of the seriously ill patient, one sees a somewhat more variable picture. There are many physicians and nurses who see the emotional, social and psychological ramifications of illness as deserving of their attention. Their interest in the whole patient and all of his problems keeps faith with the finest traditions of medicine. But the ability of professional caregivers in this respect varies immensely from individual to individual. Within the hospital and within society at large there are available today many support systems for dealing with psychological and social problems which were not available in the past; there are social work departments, counseling services and financial assistance organizations of various types. However, a number of factors have tended to make institutions and individuals less willing and able to attend to the emotional, social and psychological problems of the seriously ill patient and his family.

All of the above matters relate to the seriously ill patient and his family whether or not death is impending. The fact of impending death introduces the whole panorama of problems related to death, separation and loss. Superimposed now on the fear of pain and discomfort arising from illness are fears about dying and about death. Ours has been characterized as a death-denying and a youth-oriented society; in large measure, these charges are doubtless true. Ours is an urbanized society which has lost touch with the cycles of nature and has come to expect medical science to conquer all disease. These attitudes toward death have unquestionably helped shape both personal reaction and public policy toward death. In any event, for the dying patient and his family, problems in dealing with death are added to the medical and non-medical problems they face.

In recent years, there has been increasing attention to death and dying which hopefully will, in the long run, provide some practical results in the way in which people approach death. The seminal work of Elizabeth Kübler-Ross (1969) sharpened the focus on the process of dying which was characteristic of the decade of the 1970s. Brim (1970) and Horan and Mall (1977) have viewed from a broad perspective the matter of dealing with the dying. Ramsay (1970) and others have explored the ethical issues related to our attitudes toward death. Noyes (1971) and Dunphy (1976) have looked critically at the clinical aspects of care of the dying. There has been recognition within medical schools that medical students should be taught about death and dying (Barton et al., 1972). In the medical and non-medical literature, terminal disease, dying and death are being addressed far more frequently and far more perceptively than they were a few years ago.

Nonetheless, there remain a number of factors that interfere with making the dying process as comfortable as possible. These problems are as real as they are obvious; their effects can be seen daily in graphic, personal terms. For example, they lead often to one of two medical approaches to the terminally ill patient which, though different, are not necessarily mutually exclusive. At one extreme there may be a "nothing further can be done" approach in which semantic confusion occurs between being able to do nothing further *about the tumor* and being able to do nothing further *for the patient;* these are two very different things. At the other extreme, there is the frantic utilization of multiple modalities of anti-tumor therapy and aggressive life support systems in a vain effort to "do something"; there is a confusion between what *can* be done and what *should* be done.

Similarly, professional caregivers and families alike, because of difficulties related to the acceptance of impending death, find themselves with no meaningful way in which to relate to the patient and to each other. A number of unhappy scenarios may result. The most common is probably the closing of all lines of communication so that the patient and his family see the caregivers as cold and heartless and the caregivers see the patient's family as unconcerned. Another common pattern is that in which the caregivers feel helpless, but see the patient's family as demanding and guilt-ridden. In summary, the criticisms of terminal care which we hear most frequently from dying patients and their families are the unnecessary prolongation of life, ineffective control of symptoms, lack of emotional support and fragmentation of caregiving responsibility.

Before approaching the matter of methods for dealing with these problems of terminal illness, we must establish an operational definition. In a sense, each of us is terminally ill from the day he is born. (Silver (1980) has, however, quite correctly described this concept as "excessively lugubrious and . . . not workable.") In the context in which it is used here, terminal illness is defined as the existence of a malignant tumor for which anti-tumor therapy does not offer a reasonable possibility of cure.

It is evident that all of the problems identified above in dealing with terminal illness are compounded by the fact that, as defined, the terminally ill are not a homogeneous group. They are highly individual. Each brings to his terminal illness a tumor of specific type and extent, individual manifestations of his tumor and individual attitudes toward his disease, his family and his impending death. Furthermore, all of these factors are dynamic, not static; they are constantly changing. It is not surprising, therefore, that the provision of optimal care for the dying patient is difficult and is deserving of our most thoughtful attention and strenuous effort.

Objectives in the Care of Terminal Illness

The logical place to begin in the design of a program for the care of the terminally ill is with the objectives of such a program. What is it we would like to accomplish in the care of the patient dying of malignant disease?

The articulation of practical, helpful objectives in the care of terminal illness is not a simple task. Differences of opinion regarding definitions and substantive matters create difficulty. It is very easy to become entangled in a web of controversy while simply trying to identify the principal purposes of a program.

Considerable disagreement has occurred over the phrase "death with dignity" as a goal of programs for the care of terminal illness (e.g., Vanderpool, 1978). The term "graceful" has been suggested as a more appropriate description than "dignified" as the way in which most of us wish to die. Though the distinction may seem trivial, the controversy itself perhaps suggests some deep differences in the way in which people think about optimal handling of the dying process. As a physician, the author's bias has always been toward "comfort" and the phrase we use at Church Hospital is "toward a gentler dying."

In examining the objectives of good palliative care for the terminally ill, attention must obviously be directed both to the *quantity* of life and to the *quality* of life. Because both are important, the two must be balanced. It is the thesis of this book that there are presently available techniques that can help achieve this balance and thus make terminal illness a more comfortable experience for the patient and his family. Yet we must recognize that there are very real problems in approaching both quantity and quality of life. In the patient with advanced cancer, quantity can be easily measured in terms of days, weeks or months, but often we simply do not have available the information that will tell us how various options in treatment will effect the quantity of life. Furthermore, predictions of quantity of life without therapy are at best crude. Quality of life presents the problem of not being measurable. Factors influencing the quality of life are not only highly individual for each patient but are extremely subjective.

It is easy to set the provision of a maximum quantity and quality of life with an appropriate balance of the two as an overall goal in the care of the terminally ill. However, we would deceive ourselves if we did not recognize that for a particular patient with disseminated breast cancer, for example, we cannot predict with accuracy what effect the administration of a given program of chemotherapy will have on her life expectancy. Nor can we determine in advance the degree of discomfort she will perceive; we certainly cannot determine for her whether she would prefer three months of uncomfortable life to an earlier, more comfortable death. Even the patient may have difficulty assigning priorities to the relief and avoidance of various symptoms of her disease and its therapy. Such are the vagaries of advanced malignant disease and its handling, but in any program for the care of the terminally ill we, with the help of the patient and family, are going to have to make these decisions.

With these reservations in mind, the following are suggested objectives for a program for the care of the terminally ill:

1. *Provide the finest available medical care for the patient's medical problems.* This means treatment directed both at control of the patient's disease

and optimal relief of his symptoms. Treatment of the underlying disease must be undertaken with the recognition that, by definition, cure is not possible, but that control of the disease may contribute materially to palliation.

2. *Provide, for the patient and his family, appropriate understanding of the nature of the patient's situation and psychological support to both in dealing with the illness and with impending death.* What constitutes "appropriate" understanding will be highly individual for each patient.

3. *Provide appropriate spiritual support to the patient and family in dealing with the philosophic and religious aspects of the illness and impending death.*

4. *Provide assistance to the patient and family in dealing with interpersonal, social and financial problems.*

5. *Render patient care in the optimal setting for the particular circumstances.* For some patients all care will be in an institution, for others all care can best be rendered at home and for the remainder a combination of the two will be necessary.

6. *Provide certain valuable program characteristics such as continuity, comprehensiveness and adaptability to individual circumstances.* There are many facets of this objective. Care of the seriously ill tends, because of technology and specialization, to be fragmented; this fragmentation has a number of negative consequences. A corollary of the need for continuity is the need for 24-hour availability of personnel. "Programs" by their very nature tend to be somewhat inflexible and special attention needs to be devoted to the matter of adaptability to individual circumstances.

7. *Provide a setting for research into the care of the terminally ill.* We have much to learn if we are going to do things better.

8. *Provide for ongoing education in the care of the terminally ill.* This means education both for those whose primary concern is dealing with the dying patient and education for others who may at one time or another be involved with the care of the terminally ill.

9. *Have a positive impact on the remainder of the health care system.* As noted, some of the problems which plague the terminally ill and their families are also very real problems for other patients and their families. Hopefully, as we learn more about the proper handling of terminal illness, we will learn things which can be applied in general medical care. Even failing this objective, programs for the care of the terminally ill should not be disruptive of the remainder of health care system and should integrate well with it.

10. *Be financially feasible.* All of these objectives may not be equally vital and achievable, and they are not listed in order of importance. As with the other

objectives, there are problems of definition (is it cost effective?) and sub-stantive problems (how do you get reimbursed for it?), but we would be unrealistic if we did not include this as an objective of a program for the care of the terminally ill.

There is one special caution with respect to these objectives. They are targets toward which we must aim as we develop programs for the terminally ill. No program will reach every objective at its inception; he who waits for a perfect program will have no program at all.

There is one final concern before beginning to look at the hospice concept as a response to the needs of the dying patient. As individuals and programs emerge to deal with problems, there is often a tendency for others to let up a little in the belief that the burden has now been fully and safely taken up. It is important to remember that palliative care is a responsibility, not just of those who are directly involved in its delivery, but also of the clinician whose primary responsibility is the provision of curative treatment to cancer patients. It is he who must make the often difficult decision that there is no longer a reasonable hope of cure and thus commit the patient to a program of palliative care. However, his responsibility begins even before this. In certain forms of malignancy (for example, esophageal and pancreatic cancer), the potential for cure is often extremely limited even when the patient is seen early in the course of his disease. In the initial planning of treatment for such patients, the prudent clinician is careful that in providing a slim chance of cure he does not materially reduce the potential for adequate palliation. The consequences of an unwise choice of curative therapy can some-times be a greater barrier to "a gentler dying" than is the underlying malig-nancy.

Hospice Care as a Response

For a number of reasons, hospice care is somewhat difficult to define. This is in part because the term "hospice" dates back to the Middle Ages and over the years has had different meanings. Furthermore, present day hospice care is char-acterized by its diversity. Nonetheless, the modern hospice has certain distinctive features and, if it cannot be defined concisely, it can at least be described. Hospice care is a comprehensive program of management which offers an opportunity to provide palliative care for terminally ill patients. Its multidiscipli-nary approach is designed to relieve the patient's symptoms and to provide sup-port to both the patient and his family. It is care that can be rendered in any one of a number of settings: the patient's home, a nursing home, a free-standing hospice unit or a hospital. Although most hospice programs have focused primar-ily upon terminal illness from malignant disease, many have provided care to other types of patients, such as those with progressive neurological diseases, including multiple sclerosis and amyotrophic lateral sclerosis.

In medieval times, a hospice was a way station for travellers; in this sense, the adoption of the term for a program for the care of the terminally ill is quite fitting. However, there are obviously some problems with its use. Before the term was adopted by programs for the dying, it had already been used by other types of institutions such as convalescent homes and facilities for the care of the mentally ill. In addition, the term possesses a religious connotation to which some have taken exception. Some programs that clearly are hospices in the functional sense have for these reasons adopted other names, such as "palliative care unit" or "home." Although the term may lack clarity, its use is widely accepted and there does not appear to be an alternative that is both simple and accurate.

The lack of precision of the term "hospice" has created some practical problems. It is not reasonable to seek a copyright on the term; in turn, this creates difficulties in certification and accreditation, as there can be no restriction on the use of the term.

At this point it would be well to observe that the word "hospice" is presently used as both a noun and adjective. The noun "hospice" possesses different meanings. It is used as part of the title of certain convalescent and residential homes that are only incidently involved in the care of the terminally ill. These institutions have usually possessed the name hospice for many years and, except coincidently, are not involved in the use of present day hospice principles in palliative care. An example is the Stella Mara Hospice near Baltimore. "Hospice" is also used as a noun to describe the type of care for the terminally ill that is the subject of this book. But even here it has several meanings. Sometimes it is used to describe a place or physical facility, such as Hospice Inc. of Connecticut. Sometimes it is used to describe a program that has little or no exclusive location, such as the Church Hospital hospice. Sometimes it is used to encompass the entire approach to terminal illness that is based upon the principles of hospice care, as in "hospice is an idea whose time has come." As an adjective used to modify nouns such as care, program, concept, movement and approach, hospice almost invariably denotes management of terminal illness.

In tracing the history of hospice care, it is difficult to know precisely where to begin. One might start with medieval institutions which were termed hospices or with institutions devoted to the care of the terminally ill, whether designated as hospices or not. Alternatively, one might consider the initial hospices to be individuals, institutions or programs which used some of the principles associated with present day hospice care. The early history of hospice is intertwined in part with that of hospitals, for the latter were at one time largely places for the dying poor. The modern day hospice program has its origin in the pioneering work of Cicely Saunders in the care of the terminally ill, which led her to open St. Christopher's Hospice in Syndenham, England, in 1967. The concept spread rapidly throughout England with the opening of many hospices. These were almost exclusively free-standing units separate from hospitals.

Hospice care came to North America in January 1975 with the opening of the Palliative Care Unit at the Royal Victoria Hospital in Montreal under the direction of Dr. Balfour Mount (Mount, 1976b). This very successful prototype program is a hospital-based unit. At about the same time an imaginative, industrious and pioneering group at New Haven was founding Hospice Incorporated of Connecticut (Lack and Buckingham, 1978); this was a free-standing unit which began with home care before it possessed a physical facility. As in England, the hospice concept has caught on in North America; there are now many hospices in various stages of operation and planning throughout the United States and Canada. Because of problems with definition and data gathering and because the situation is dynamic, it is difficult to say precisely how many hospice programs are in existence at any given moment. The Comptroller General of the United States (1979) has reported that in November 1978 there were 59 operating hospices in the United States. Cohen (1979) lists more than 200 hospices in different stages of development in this country.

The transplantation of hospice care from the United Kingdom to the United States has required some modification in hospice organization. In addition to obvious general social and cultural differences between the two countries, there are some very important differences in the medical care systems. England, of course, has a compulsory national health insurance system which the United States does not. An even more important difference, however, relates to the way in which physicians are organized to deliver health care in the two countries. In England there are two categories of physicians; these are general practitioners who work strictly on an outpatient basis and specialists (consultants) who work strictly within hospitals. Every citizen is not only assigned to a general practitioner but also has a district nurse. This is a vastly different health care delivery system from that in the United States and this difference has had an impact as hospice care has come to America.

There has been concomitant development of hospice programs around the world. In June 1980 the author was privileged to attend the International Hospice Conference in London. At that celebration of its ''bar-mitzvah'' by St. Christopher's, there were representatives of hospices in 17 countries, including three representatives from behind the Iron Curtain.

Cohen (1979) traces the origin and development of hospice programs. Stoddard (1978) also provides a colorful look at the history of hospices and many of the personalities who have been important in its development.

Although all are committed to providing palliative care for the terminally ill, hospices throughout the United States have taken various forms and have had various criteria for the admission of patients. Basically, they have been of several organizational types:

1. Home care only.
2. Free-standing hospice unit, usually with provision of home care.

3. Hospital-based program, usually with provision of home care.
   a) Discrete unit within the hospital.
   b) No discrete unit within the hospital.
      Within this subcategory, several different approaches have been employed. Some programs have utilized, "swing beds" on one nursing unit and others have used a "scatter bed" approach throughout the hospital. Both of these systems in effect utilize a symptom control team which may either serve in a consultant capacity to the attending physician or take primary responsibility for the care of the patient.

It must be emphasized that the distinction between these several organizational types is not always clear-cut. There are numerous variations in the types listed. For example, there are some free-standing units that are hospital-affiliated; in other words, the physical facility for care of the terminally ill is outside of the hospital, but the program there is in some measure co-ordinated with in-hospital care. Although it is not absolute, the classification used here is useful in beginning our look at hospice care.

The diversity of hospice care is evident; although it has created some problems, unquestionably, it has also been one of the strengths of hospice care. It has permitted the development of hospices under circumstances in which a more standardized format would have been stifling. In addition, it has encouraged the type of innovation that is essential to growth.

Furthermore, through their diversity, hospices have many things in common. Their orientation is humanistic in the sense of concern for the well-being of the patient and his family. They are holistic in the sense of directing attention to "the whole patient" and drawing upon the whole armamentarium of medical care through the use of a multidisciplinary team. Their focus is upon life and living rather than upon death and dying. They view death as a natural part of life, but as one which, like birth, can be made easier by the provision of some help.

These shared characteristics, together with some common approaches and techniques, are what is included under the term "hospice" as it is applied to the care of the terminally ill patient and his family.

The National Hospice Organization (NHO) was formed in 1977 and is incorporated in Washington, D.C. It is composed of various categories of institutional and individual members and is governed by a board of directors. Membership is open to individuals and institutions interested in hospice care, but voting membership is restricted to incorporated providers of hospice care and regional and state-wide hospice organizations. The purposes of the NHO include the exchange of information between hospice groups, the provision of information about hospice care to the public and the establishment and maintenance of standards of hospice care.

Although no federal legislation dealing specifically with hospices has yet been enacted, the Department of Health, Education and Welfare has taken notice of the development of hospice programs. It has, among other actions, designated certain hospice programs as pilot projects for the purposes of studying mechanisms of reimbursement for hospice care. A number of state legislatures have passed bills and resolutions of various types dealing with care of the terminally ill generally and hospice care specifically. In Maryland, for example, a Hospice Care Reimbursement Study Commission has been established under the auspices of the state legislature to determine what types of services beneficial to the terminally ill and their families are and are not presently available and how the insurance industry and the state's medical assistance program shall approach the provision of needed forms of insurance coverage. Actions taken in other states range from the establishment of hospice pilot projects to acts defining hospice care and including hospices in the state's certificate of need and facility licensing laws. In various ways, government at different levels and locales has taken cognizance of the existence of hospice care.

There are some additional matters related to hospices in general which deserve comment at this point.

As has been pointed out, the word hospice has been used as an adjective before a number of nouns including movement, concept and philosophy. In a sense there are and have been all of these things, although as a surgeon the author finds the phrase "hospice movement" somewhat awkward and confusing. We have reached the point where hospice programs are just as much a reality as are open heart surgery programs. Granting the obvious differences, the latter also developed without an "open heart surgery movement." Perhaps the term "movement" reflects the relatively greater involvement of individuals outside the medical field in the development of hospice programs. This initiative and support is welcome and essential. However, there is an aspect of this issue that raises some concern. Although hospice care depends upon a multidisciplinary approach, utilizes families and volunteers in imaginative ways and requires support from outside the health care team, hospice care in particular and medical care in general will suffer if hospice care becomes separated from medical care. To meet its full potential, hospice care must be a medical program. To the extent that a hospice movement stimulates and supports a medical program of hospice care for the terminally ill, our society will be enriched. However, a movement growing outside of the medical care system can pose serious dangers. The ways in which hospice care can be interlocked into our health care system are multiple and can be adapted to local circumstances. It would be regrettable if medical and non-medical people failed to co-operate in providing optimal care for the terminally ill.

It has been argued that hospice care is not a new development, but rather a return to old values. There is little to be gained from exploration of this argument. Surely hospice care is founded upon the finest traditions of medical care and man's concern for his fellow man. Clearly it utilizes some techniques that date back many years. However, as is often the case with worthwhile advances, it represents some new applications of old knowledge. The successful use of a broad-based multidisciplinary team is not unique to hospice care, but no one can deny that this approach has immensely enlarged the scope of our capacity to deal with the terminally ill.

It is important to point out that hospice care programs have not provided all of the answers to the problems of caring for the terminally ill. As with many worthwhile endeavors, hospice care has raised more questions than it has answered. However, pertinent questions lead to progress. This may seem trite and pedantic, but its practical importance to hospice programs cannot be over-emphasized. Unrealistic expectations on the part of patients, families and hospice workers have probably led to more unhappy consequences than any other single factor in hospice care. It is important to recognize and accept the fact that the best of hospice care is not going to make every death beautiful and easy. The zeal of hospice workers and the enthusiasm of surviving family members have contributed immensely to the success of hospice care, but they must be tempered by an understanding that serious illness and death have unpleasant features which cannot be overcome by any program designed and operated by human beings.

References

Alsop, S.: *Stay of Execution*. Philadelphia, Lippincott (1973)

Barton, D.; Flexner, J.M.; van Eys, J.; Scott, C.E.: Death and Dying: A Course for Medical Students. J Med Educ Vol. 47, 945 (1972)

Brim, O.G.: *The Dying Patient*. New York, N.Y. The Russell Sage Foundation (1970)

Cohen, K.P.: *Hospice: Prescription for Terminal Care*. Germantown, Md. Aspen Press (1979)

Comptroller General: Report to the Congress of the United States. HRD 79–50 (March 6, 1979)

Dunphy, J.E.: Annual Discourse—On Caring for the Patient With Cancer. N Engl J Med Vol. 295, 313 (1976)

Gunther, J.: *Death Be Not Proud*. New York, N.Y. Harper Brothers (1949)

Horan, D.J.; Mall, D.: *Death, Dying and Euthanasia*. Washington, D.C. University Publications of America (1977)

Lack, S.A.; Buckingham, R.W.: *First American Hospice*. New Haven, Conn. Hospice Inc. (1978)

Mount, B.M.: The Problem of caring for the dying in a general hospital; the palliative care unit as a possible solution. Can Med Assoc J Vol. 115, 119 (1976a)

Mount, B.M.: *Palliative Care Service: October 1976 Report*. Montreal Royal Victoria Hospital/McGill University (1976b)

Noyes, R.: The Care and Management of the Dying. Arch Intern Med Vol. 128, 299 (1971)

Ramsey, P.: *The Patient as a Person*. New Haven, Conn. Yale University Press (1970)

Kubler-Ross, E.: *On Death and Dying*. New York, N.Y. Mac Millan (1969)

Ryder, C.F.; Ross, D.M.: Terminal Care—Issues and Alternatives. Public Health Rep, Vol. 92, 20 (1977)

Silver, R.T.: The Dying Patient: A Clinician's View. Am J Med, Vol. 68, 473 (1980)

Stoddard, S.: *The Hospice Movement*. Briarcliff Manor, N.Y., Stein and Day (1978)

Vanderpool, H.Y.: The Ethics of Terminal Care. JAMA, Vol. 239, 850 (1978)

2. The Church Hospital Hospice Experience

Description of the Program

The hospice care program at Church Hospital has developed gradually over the last several years. It is devoted to patient care and education and research in the treatment of terminal illness due to malignant disease.

Church Hospital is a private 310 bed urban general hospital with an active medical staff of approximately 100 physicians. Its major clinical services are Medicine, Surgery and Gynecology. It does not have Pediatric, Obstetrical or Psychiatric services and offers no residency training programs. Its approximately 10,000 admissions per year result in an occupancy rate of just under 90%.

The hospice care program at the hospital was first proposed by the hospital chaplain, Reverend Paul Dawson, who interested key members of the medical and hospital staff of various departments. This group studied the experience of hospice programs in the United Kingdom and North America; it became convinced that a hospice program at Church Hospital would meet a need and would be feasible. The concept was very carefully presented to the medical staff, the hospital management and the board of directors to obtain their concurrence. A program specifically designed for Church Hospital was then developed and approved by each of these groups. The program was begun gradually by incorporating various features of hospice care, such as measures for pain control and the provision of emotional support, into the care of terminally ill patients. Subsequently, the decision was made to place all hospice inpatients in swing beds on one nursing unit. It is from that move in December of 1977 that we date the formal initiation of our program. Because even today there is no designated hospice area on that unit, our hospice is a *program,* not a *place,* and the date of its true beginning is difficult to pinpoint. By the very nature of the state of the art of the management of terminal illness, it is a developing program. The hospital's home health program, which handles both hospice and non-hospice patients, was certified in the spring of 1978.

The Church Hospital hospice program, which is a hospital-based program without a discrete physical facility, is under the direction of a medical staff committee which establishes policy and oversees the program. The committee is composed primarily of physicians. The author is chairman of the committee; the hospice physician is a member, as are three additional members of the medical staff who have no other immediate connection with the program. There is representation from the other disciplines involved in the hospice program, including nursing and social work. There is cross-representation on the Home Care Committee which oversees the home care program.

The Committee meets regularly and reports to the Medical Executive Committee, which in turn is responsible to the hospital Board of Directors. The hospice committee has drawn up, and periodically makes appropriate revisions of, a hospice care program manual which articulates guidelines for operation of the program. In essence, the organization and implementation of the hospice is similar to that of other specialized patient care programs within the hospital, such as the hyperalimentation and cardiac rehabilitation programs.

A hospice physician, whose background is in family practice, is employed part-time. He supervises the day-to-day operation of the program and serves as the attending physician for many of the patients in the program. In his absence, the chairman of the Hospice Committee or one of the other physician members of the committee takes over his duties.

Hospice care at Church Hospital is designed to serve patients of members of the Church Hospital medical staff. A few other patients referred by physicians in the community or by physicians on the staff of the Oncology Center at the Johns Hopkins Hospital, which is located one block away, are accepted. On rare occasions a patient is accepted into the program on his own initiative or that of his family without physician referral. Although there is no rigid limit on the number of patients in the program at any one time, the demand for hospice services is considerable; at times it is necessary to accept patients in accordance with a priority listing.

Guidelines for admission to the hospice care program are as follows:

1. The patient must be terminally ill from a malignant disease. Terminal illness is defined as that situation in which anti-tumor therapy does not offer a reasonable possibility of cure, as determined by the patient's attending physician in consultation with the hospice physician.

2. Life expectancy should be more than 5 days but in most instances less than 6 months.

3. It is desirable but not necessary that the patient be referred by a physician and that the patient's attending physician give consent for entry into the program.

4. The patient must reside within a reasonable distance of the hospital and must have at least one involved family member or friend who will accept responsibility for care-giving. An exception is made if, on the basis of his disease,

there is no reasonable prospect that the patient will ever be suitable for home care and if life expectancy is short.

5. Patients and their families are accepted into the program only with the full understanding and acceptance of this mode of treatment.

6. Corollaries:
    a) Patients with severe symptom control problems shall be given priority consideration.
    b) Admission to the inpatient unit is limited to patients whose needs are such that they cannot be met by home care.

From the first the Church Hospital Hospice Care Program was, for practical reasons, open only to patients terminally ill from advanced malignancy. It was recognized that the demand for a hospice program would be substantial, but that our capacity would be limited. The experience and interest of our medical staff in malignant disease were the principal factors in making the decision to limit the program to such patients.

Although there might in some instances be disagreement as to whether a particular patient has reached the point where anti-tumor therapy offers a reasonable possibility of cure, as a practical matter this has seldom been an issue for our hospice care program. There is obviously an element of self-selection in this; by the time the attending physician refers the patient, he has already reached the conclusion that the patient is terminally ill. One of our hopes for the future is that physicians will refer patients at an earlier stage of their terminal illness. If this happens, we may begin to see more patients for whom there is some question whether all curative measures have been exhausted. Church Hospital has an effective, functioning Tumor Board in which internists, surgeons, oncologists and radiation therapists participate. Its recommendations, although not binding, are very helpful to the attending physician in determining whether or not there is a reasonable possibility of cure for his patient.

Even though duration of life in most patients with advanced malignancy is impossible to predict with any degree of accuracy, a guideline relating to life expectancy is included in order to distribute the limited resources of the program among those patients with the greatest prospect of benefiting from it. Patients who live only a day or two after entry into the program gain little from it and the extent to which their families can profit is limited. Most patients with more than 6 months' life expectancy are relatively free of symptoms and are able to cope with their situation satisfactorily without all of the features of hospice care. Their admission is deferred until they become symptomatic. Recognizing the vagaries of prediction of life expectancy and the fact that some with life expectancy outside the designated limits will benefit materially from the hospice program, Guideline 2 is often relaxed.

Circumstances do occur in which a patient makes direct application for entry into the program without referral from his attending physician. If it seems that the patient is otherwise a candidate for the program, every reasonable effort is made to secure the attending physician's agreement to entry. If, however, this cannot be obtained and it appears on the basis of available evidence that the patient would profit from the program, the case is considered on its individual merits.

Our program does not presently have an established relationship with an intermediate care facility. Consequently, no patient with a life expectancy of more than several weeks and the prospect of being sent home is taken into the program unless he resides within a reasonable distance of the hospital and there is an identifiable care-giver in the home. Without this provision, the program would be confronted with patients who do not require care in an acute general hospital but for whom there would be no other way to provide hospice care. This guideline is relaxed in special circumstances; in such instances, an effort is made to continue as much hospice care as possible through appropriate individual arrangements with a nursing home. We are presently in the process of attempting to fill this gap in our hospice care program through the development of a formal ongoing relationship with a nursing home facility. This would open our program to certain patients who are now excluded, as it would assure the availability of hospice measures at all three levels of care: acute in-hospital, intermediate and home care.

The matter of what constitutes "full understanding" of the situation and the issue of informed consent are delicate, complex and highly individualized problems. Our handling of this topic is presented in Chapter 3.

Inquiries regarding patient referral to the hospice program are directed to the Home Care Office, where basic information about the patient and his status is obtained. Initial screening is carried out in this department. It is also through this office that the patient and his family are given information about the program. If the patient appears to the home health director to meet the guidelines, the application is referred to the clinical nurse practitioner on the hospice inpatient unit and to the hospice physician; together they make the final determination regarding acceptance of the patient. If necessary, they place him on the priority list. Ordinarily, a decision can be made within a few hours of referral.

It should be mentioned that the decision to utilize this sequence in dealing with applications for admission to the program is based strictly upon the personnel and support facilities (such as secretarial assistance) available in the hospital. This point is simply illustrative of the need to adapt a hospice care program to local circumstances.

Sometimes, when an attending physician suggests entry into the hospice program, patients and their families are uncertain or reluctant. There are a number of reasons for this. It may be a manifestation of denial, the patient and family may be coping well with the situation or there may be uncertainty about the nature of hospice care. In such circumstances, the patient and his family are given an opportunity to discuss the hospice program thoroughly with members of the hospice staff; following this discussion a decision can be made. One decision may be to defer entry into the program. An occasional patient who enters the program while quite ill will improve enough so that he and his family do not feel the need of ongoing full-fledged hospice care. In that situation, the patient is placed temporarily on inactive status and his case is made active again when the situation warrants.

When the decision has been made to accept the patient into the hospice care program, the referring physician is required to complete some basic information forms (Figures 1–3). These are usually supplemented by discussion with the hospice physician and the clinical nurse practitioner.

Once the patient is formally accepted, it is understood that the care given will be symptomatic and palliative, in accordance with hospice care objectives and philosophy. Anti-tumor therapy will be utilized only insofar as it contributes to palliation.

For those patients who are referred to the program from outside the Church Hospital medical staff, the hospice physician becomes the patient's attending physician in the hospice program. An important feature of the Church Hospital program, however, is that members of the medical staff of the hospital referring patients to the program have the option of turning the patient over to the hospice physician or of continuing as the patient's attending physician, utilizing the hospice physician as consultant. In either event, all of the facilities of the program are available to the patient and his family. This approach has the advantage of making the program appealing to different types of physicians. A referring physician who has known and followed the patient for many years is able to retain that relationship. On the other hand, a referring physician whose contact with the patient has been relatively limited is able to refer the patient to an environment where he knows the patient's needs will be met. The potential problems in such an approach are evident. It is theoretically possible that an attending physician with little knowledge of the principles and practice of hospice care can elect to retain responsibility for his patient. In actual practice, a fine balance of diplomacy, education and perseverance on the part of the hospice staff has kept this from being a serious or frequent problem. The value of this option on the part of the referring physician in terms of gaining medical staff acceptance of the program and in terms of controlling the work load of the hospice physician cannot be underestimated.

All hospice care inpatients are placed on one 50-bed general medical-surgical unit which consists of one- and two-bed rooms. Within this nursing unit there are no beds set aside for hospice patients; such patients are more or less randomly distributed in accordance with bed availability. In other words, a bed occupied today by a hospice care patient may be occupied tomorrow by a non-hospice patient; within any two-bed room, there may be one hospice patient and one non-hospice patient.

The staff on this nursing unit consists of the usual nursing staff found on a

CHURCH HOSPITAL CORPORATION
BALTIMORE, MARYLAND

HOSPICE MEDICAL FORM

A COPY OF THE MEDICAL SUMMARY SHOULD BE SENT TO THE HOME CARE OFFICE.

1. From what disease is patient suffering?   1._____

2. Duration?   2._____

3. Primary focus of disease?   3._____
    (Please specify location as closely as possible.) _____

4. Secondary deposits with sites?   4._____

5. Has patient undergone any operation?   5._____

    (a) If so, where?   (a)_____

    (b) What was the nature, date and   (b)_____
        findings? (full details)   _____
                                                      _____

6. Has patient undergone any irradiation?   6._____
    If so, state region of body irradiated   _____
    and dates.   _____

7. Has patient had any cytotoxic or hormone   7._____
    therapy? Please state details.   _____
                                                      _____

8. Is the patient currently on any of the following, 8.
    please state dosage in all cases.

    (a) Analgesics?   (a)_____

    (b) Steroids?   (b)_____

    (c) Hormones?   (c)_____

    (d) Tranquilizers or sedatives?   (d)_____

    (e) Any other drugs?   (e)_____

9. Has she/he any drug idiosyncrasies?   9._____
                                                      _____

10. What is the estimated expectation of   10._____
    life in weeks?

Figure 1a.

11. What is the present condition of the
     patient:

    (a) Pain?

    (b) Other severe symptoms?
        Anorexia_____
        Nausea_____
        Vomiting_____
        Dysphagia_____
        Bleeding_____
        Edema_____
        Discharges_____
        Cough_____
        Sleep_____
        Dyspnea_____
        Bedsores_____

    (c) Mental State?

    (d) Incontinence of bladder or bowels?

    (e) Activity level?

11.

(a)_____

(b)_____
   _____
   _____
   _____

(c)_____

(d)_____
   _____

(e)_____

12. What has the patient been told about his/
    her illness?

    _____
    _____
    _____

13. Family understand the attitude?

    _____
    _____

    _____
    _____

SIGNATURE OF DOCTOR

_____ Date of Signing _____

Address _____ Tel. No. _____

Figure 1b.

Phone: 732-4730		**CHURCH HOSPITAL CORPORATION** BALTIMORE, MARYLAND	Type	☐ Initial
Ext. 357-358-359		**REFERRAL FOR HOME HEALTH SERVICES**	of Request	☐ Change of Ord. ☐ Renewal

Patient's Name		Soc. Sec. #		Phone No.		Birth Date	Age	Sex	Race	M/S
Street Address		City		State	Zip Code	Regis. Date	Health Plan Estab.		Started Care	
Service	P/T	F/C	Payment Source							
Primary Care Taker		Relationship		Phone No.		Address				
Next of Kin		Relationship		Phone No.		Address				
Guarantor		Relationship		Phone No.		Address				
Name of Qualifying Institution		Address					Verified Dates of Stay			
Other Ins. Plan & Policy #	Group No.	Effective Date		Expiration Date		Name of Policy Holder			P/H Birth Date	
Medicare No./Health Insurance Claim No.		Medicaid Number				Date of Issue	Expiration Date			
Attending Physician		Address				Dr. No.		Phone No.		
Medical Alert						Prognosis				
Diagnosis								Related to Employment?		
Secondary Diagnosis						Estimate of Inpatient days saved				

Est. of patient's need for Services — Weeks Visits per week_____ Months	Therapeutic Goals:
Services: Skilled Nursing ☐ PT ☐ ST ☐ Ancillary: SW ☐ Nutr ☐ HH Aide ☐	Diagnosis known by patient _____ Diagnosis known by family _____
Physician's Orders and Treatment: **Medication ordered:** (Specify dose, route of administration and frequency)	Activities: Bed rest _____ Activity Limitations Chair _____ Stairs _____ As tolerated _____
	Diet _____ (Type)
	Copy to Patient Instructed
	Supplies/equipment
	Baseline Vital Signs
	Assessment: Nursing, Physical Therapy, Social Services
Other Orders, Treatments	
	Discharge Planner Signature Date

From: (Agency, Physician) Please Print	Medical Supervision at home provided by
Full Name _____	Name _____ (Physician or Clinic)
Address _____	Address _____
Phone _____	Phone _____

CERTIFICATION AND RECERTIFICATION STATEMENT: I certify that the above-named patient is under my care, is homebound except when receiving outpatient services, requires skilled nursing care or therapy on an intermittent basis as specified in the established plans of care and is periodically reviewed by me.

Physician's Signature	Date

Home Health

1-08036 (Rev. 1-80) 1M W.P. 1-80   **CHART COPY**

Figure 2.

←

CHURCH HOSPITAL CORPORATION
BALTIMORE, MARYLAND

ORDERED		DOCTOR'S ORDERS AND SIGNATURES	CARDED BY	ORDER COM-PLETED
DATE	HOUR			
		ROUTINE HOSPICE ADMISSION ORDERS		
		1. Defer weights		
		2. Vital Signs only at:		
		3. I&O		
		4. No blood work or tests unless ordered by physician		
		5. Physical Therapy: Yes ___ No ___		
		6. Aqueous morphine ___ mgm q ___ hrs.		
		Awaken for dose: Yes ___ No ___		
		Other analgesic:		
		7. Antiemetics: Compazine liquid ___ cc q ___ hrs.		
		Compazine suppositories ___ mg q ___ hrs.		
		No NG tube unless ordered by physician.		
		8. Antidepressants:		
		9. Tranquilizers:		
		10. Appetite stimulants –		
		Alcohol before or after meals		
		11. Bowel stimulants		
		PRN SS enema ___, Fleet enema ___, oil retention enema ___		
		check for fecal impaction q week ___		
		12. Antidiarrheal:		
		13. Sedatives:		
		14. Expectorants:		
		15. Cough suppressants:		
		16. Dyspnea: PRN O_2 ___ liters per min.		
		17. Antibiotics:		
		18. Foley or Texas catheter:		
		19. Decubiti prevention		
		20. No I.V. unless ordered		
		21. Diet		
		22. Activity		

1-00100 (Rev. 8/79) 20M W.P. 6/80   **DOCTOR'S ORDER SHEET**   CHART COPY

Figure 3.

general medical-surgical floor; these are head nurse, assistant head nurse, clinical nurse practitioners, staff nurses, aides and clerical personnel. Hospital departments such as social work and physical therapy assign staff members to serve this nursing unit as they do to serve other units. All of the personnel have been specially trained in hospice care and participate in continuing education programs related to hospice care. All of them, however, on any given day, are providing care for both hospice and non-hospice patients. For the reasons identified in Chapter 8, the level of staffing on this nursing unit is essentially the same as that on the other nursing units of similar size.

In addition to the normally assigned staff on the unit, there is a cadre of carefully selected and trained volunteers who work primarily with hospice patients.

On this unit standard hospital policies and regulations are relaxed for hospice patients. For example, visiting hours are unlimited, patients are encouraged to keep favorite personal items at their bedside and are allowed to have pets visit them. There is a special visitor's lounge for families of hospice patients; this includes sleeping facilities.

One of the first steps taken at Church Hospital when the decision was made to initiate a hospice program was to strengthen the existing home care program and to gain the necessary state approval for this improvement. This home health department, which consists of a director and three other visiting nurses, operates a very active home care service for all hospital patients who qualify for the service. In other words, it serves both hospice and non-hospice patients. As noted above, one of the criteria for acceptance of patients into the hospice program specifies that the location of the patient's home and the home situation will permit home care.

The determination of whether to provide care at home or in the hospital environment rests almost solely with the patient's need for an acute level of care. In some instances, families, either for emotional or physical reasons, are no longer capable of providing care. Typical reasons for admission to the hospital include intractable pain, intestinal obstruction, respiratory failure, persistent nausea and vomiting, peripheral vascular insufficiency, hemorrhage, seizures and mental confusion. Once the patient's condition has been stabilized, an effort is made to return the patient to his home.

Employing principles and practices of sound hospice care and enlisting the help of family in providing certain elements of care, it is possible for the home health staff to render terminal care of the highest quality to patients in their homes.

In addition to home health department staff, other members of the hospice team, such as social worker, physical therapist, chaplain and volunteers, are available to make home visits as needed.

Table I shows the staffing assignment breakdown with respect to inpatient-outpatient responsibilities. In point of fact, however, responsibility and involve-

Table 1.   Church Hospital Hospice Team Members' Responsibilities.

Both Inpatient and Outpatient	Inpatient Only	Outpatient Only
Hospice physician	Clinical unit nurses	Home health nurses
Social worker	Clinical nurse practitioner	Home health aides
Physical therapist	Clinical unit aides	
Chaplain	Clinical unit clerks	
Volunteers		

ment are not sharply defined. The home health department nurses frequently visit patients while they are on the inpatient unit and the inpatient personnel follow the progress of hospice patients while they are out of the hospital. The key to successful co-ordination of inpatient-outpatient care is this kind of flexibility and good communication.

In this connection it is worth noting that, with the possible exception of some of the volunteers, no one in the hospice care program is involved on a full-time basis. Everyone, including the hospice physician, inpatient nursing unit personnel, home health nurses, social workers, chaplains, etc., has other responsibilities. We feel that any disadvantages due to this lack of specialization are more than offset by the advantages of the spill-over of hospice concepts to other types of patient care. Minimization of staff stress is also a significant benefit.

As with all other aspects of patient care in the hospital, including other special programs such as hyperalimentation, the hospice care program is subject to the hospital mechanisms for quality assurance. This includes audits and other techniques of assuring the optimal quality of care. One of the advantages of a hospital-based program is that the mechanics of quality assurance are already in place; they insure an element of independent review, since the departmental audit committees are made up largely of physicians having no direct involvement in the hospice program.

Chapters 7 and 8 provide some additional details about our Home Care Department and the general organization of our hospice program.

Clinical Experience

The following material is presented in an effort to provide a picture of the clinical experience in the Church Hospital hospice program. Data have been kept on all patients entered in the program and have, from time to time, been analyzed. Our techniques of data collection and presentation are still evolving. The hospice care committee reviews basic statistical information on the program regularly.

A close look has been taken at a sample of 100 consecutive patients admitted in 1978 (Zimmerman, 1979). Breindel and Gravely (1980) have carried out a detailed statistical and financial evaluation of the Church Hospital hospice program which provides some very useful facts about our experience. The information which follows is selected from these sources.

The five most common sites of primary tumor are lung, pancreas, colon and rectum, breast and esophagus. A wide variety of other primary sites are represented; there are a few patients in whom the location of the primary tumor has never been determined.

About 10 to 12 patients per month are accepted into the Church Hospital hospice program, with considerable day-to-day and week-to-week variation. There are approximately equal numbers of males and females. They range in age from 14 to 89; roughly two thirds have been in the seventh and eighth decades of life.

The total number of hospice patients on any given day varies, but it averages 20 to 25. Of these, approximately two thirds are at home and one third are in the hospital. During one 3-month period, the inpatient hospice census ranged from 1 to 12 patients, with an average daily census of 7.1 patients. Nearly 90% of patients first enter the program while hospitalized or are immediately hospitalized upon entry into the program. Ninety-five percent of the patients spend a portion of their terminal illness in the hospital. About 80% of the patients have a single hospitalization during their stay in the program, 15% have two admissions and the remaining 5% have three or more hospitalizations.

Between 70 and 80% of all patients now entering the program spend some time at home. Approximately 50% die at home. As noted, at any given time roughly two thirds of all patients in our program are at home. Patients who are able to spend some time at home generally have a longer duration of life than those who are not.

Total length of stay in the hospice program has ranged from 1 to more than 300 days, with an average of approximately 38 days. Length of hospital stay in most samples of patients looked at has ranged from 1 to 30 days, with an average inhospital stay of approximately 12 days. For example, among 45 patients entering the program in one 3-month period, the range of inhospital length of stay was 1 to 22 days, with an average of 12.1 days. Of interest is the fact that during that 3-month period the average length of stay for all medical-surgical patients in the hospital was 10.4 days.

The home care service handles both hospice and non-hospice patients. Its average patient load at any given time is approximately 50 patients, or 14 to 16 patients per home care nurse. Of this total, approximately 15 are hospice patients. Non-hospical home care patients average about six visits per month, with each visit averaging 50 to 60 minutes. Hospice care patients receive somewhat more frequent visits, with each visit averaging close to 2 hours.

For approximately 30% of the patients entering the program, the referring physician has elected to continue as the attending physician. In the remainder, the hospice physician has served as attending physician during the patient's stay in the hospice program. There appears to be a gradual but definite increase in the percentage of patients for whom the referring physician has continued as the attending physician. Presumably, this is due to increasing familiarity with hospice principles and practice on the part of our medical staff; this is a trend which the hospice care committee has encouraged.

Approximately 80% of the patients entering the program have been referred by members of the medical staff at Church Hospital. Of the 20% who have entered the program on referral from other sources, roughly half, or 10% of the total, have been referred by the Oncology Center at Johns Hopkins Hospital.

The average cost for hospice patients in late 1979 was $174 per day or $1,920 per admission. At the same time, the cost for general medical-surgical patients was $345 per day and $3,431 per admission. In other words, hospice patients had a lower daily cost and lower average length of stay, with a resultant substantially lower per admission cost. It would appear also that the cost has been somewhat lower for patients under the care of the hospice physician than for those under the care of other staff members. In the latter group, it appears that the more familiar a patient's physician is with the hospice program and the more frequently he serves as attending physician in it, the lower the patient's costs.

Breindel and Gravely (1980) have conducted a rigorous analysis of nursing time per patient day in the Church Hospital hospice program, comparing nursing hours per patient for hospice and non-hospice patients. For hospice patients, total personnel hours per day were 7.3, of which 3.9 were nursing personnel hours and 3.4 were volunteer and family hours. During the same interval, general medical-surgical patients received 4.4 hours of total personnel time, all of it by nursing personnel.

A caveat should accompany all data on length of stay, locus in which care is provided (home versus hospital), nursing time per patient and costs. A number of factors influence these figures. The source of referral will, for example, affect the length of stay in the program. A hospital-based unit is more likely than a free-standing unit to accept patients who are acutely ill and have a short life expectancy. Hospital-based programs are therefore prone to have a higher percentage of patients in the hospital and a lower percentage of patients dying at home. Physician understanding of and confidence in a program affect the nature of referrals and thus the length of stay. Furthermore, there tend to be differences in a number of dimensions over a period of time in the early history of a program. For example, there is a changing balance between inpatient and outpatient loads during the first year or two of a program's existence as effective discharge planning is developed and as the public and medical communities adjust to the home care option.

Furthermore, there are subtle but important options in the methods of collection and analysis of data which may profoundly influence the results obtained.

For all of these reasons, one must be extremely cautious in the interpretation of data with respect to hospice programs; this is particularly true in making comparisons between different programs.

We have not analyzed information with respect to the frequency with which various symptoms or problems have occurred. One interesting and surprising point, however, is that only 58% of patients in the program have required a potent analgesic such as morphine.

Assessing the success of symptom relief in a hospice program is difficult. Since symptoms are by definition subjective, there are difficulties in measuring them and documenting changes in them. The development of techniques that will permit objective assessment of results is one of the challenges for the future, for it is in this way that we will be able to evaluate alternative approaches. It is even more difficult, of course, to assess the results of hospice team efforts in dealing with psychological and social problems and in providing spiritual support.

As a consequence we cannot speak of success rates either overall or with respect to individual problems. However, it is the uniform consensus of our hospice personnel, referring physicians and families that the net effect achieved with patients in the program has been very strongly positive. The comfort and relief brought to patients and their families by the sympathetic understanding and professional expertise of hospice workers as they deal with the psychological and practical problems of terminal illness requires no quantifying data to demonstrate the reality. With respect to symptom relief it is the author's impression that for certain symptoms, such as pain, depression, thirst and constipation, results have been extremely good; however, in the treatment of other symptoms, such as weakness, anorexia, dyspenea and dysgneusia, we have been far less successful.

Naturally, the least overall benefit was achieved by those patients who died soon after entry into the program. In retrospect, some of these patients could have been identified prior to acceptance; it is our conviction that patients with very limited life expectancy at the time of referral usually should be excluded from the program. Exceptions can occasionally be made where the benefit to family will be substantial. As familiarity with the program increases, we hope that patients will be referred to it earlier.

There have been a few patients, particularly early in our experience, who have not remained in the program until death. Some of these were patients who were accepted into the program with the understanding that their home situation would permit home care but who, because of a change of status in their home situation such as illness of the caregiver, were required to enter a nursing home where it simply was not possible to continue hospice care. Others have been patients who have decided, or for whom the family or the attending physician have decided, that further effort at curative treatment should be undertaken. As our sophistication in the provision of hospice care has increased, the frequency of dropouts has declined.

A number of observations have been made with respect to the impact of our hospice program upon non-hospice patients in the hospital and the interaction between hospice and non-hospice patients. Although there have been all types of interpersonal relationships between hospice and non-hospice patients, some positive, some negative and some neutral, it is our impression that the positive have predominated in both directions. Very seldom have we had non-hospice patients complain about the special privileges permitted hospice patients or about being in a room with a dying patient. Efforts on the part of our staff to explain the hospice program probably account in substantial measure for this. We have had a number of instances in which non-hospice patients have served an important role in the emotional support of hospice patients.

The overall effect of the hospice program on the care rendered to non-hospice patients is, of course, difficult to assess and we have at this point made no formal study. Again, it is the impression of the observers that the positive effects have predominated. There seems to be spill-over of hospice principles and practices into the care of non-hospice patients.

Church Hospital uses a patient classification system in making nursing assignments on a daily basis. This system relates staffing to severity of illness and the nursing needs of the patients. Since initiation of the hospice program, there has been no need for a major change in the number and type of nursing personnel assigned to the nursing unit on which the hospice patients are located. As this is being written, we are experimenting with the use of a modification of primary nursing care on that unit.

It is safe to say that the problems of staff stress and morale which have been experienced are, as one might anticipate with this patient mix, related primarily to the general frustrations of patient care rather than specifically to factors arising from dealing with the dying patient. In the first two years of the program, a few staff members on the inpatient nursing unit were transferred off the unit, some temporarily and some permanently, because of factors related to staff stress. Two years after assignment of all hospice patients to one nursing unit was begun, the Director of Nursing systematically interviewed each member of the nursing staff on that unit. These interviews proved very illuminating and helpful in identifying problems.

Lack and Buckingham (1978) and Walter (1979) have published extensive and detailed reports on a free-standing hospice in New Haven, Connecticut and a hospital-based hospice unit in Hayward, California. Because of organizational and methodological differences, it is difficult at present to make meaningful comparisons between hospice programs. However, the similarities between Church Hospital's hospital-based program and the one at Hayward are evident.

References

Breindel and Gravely, G.E.: *Costs of Providing a Mixed-unit Hospice Program.* Working paper, Dept. of Health Administration, Medical College of Virginia (1980)

Lack, S.A.; Buckingham, R.W.: *First American Hospice.* New Haven, Conn., Hospice Inc. (1978)

Walter, N.T.: *Hospice Pilot Project Report.* Hayward, Cal., Kaiser-Permanente (1979)

Zimmerman, J.M.: Experience with a Hospice-Care Program for the Terminally Ill. Ann Surg, Vol. 189, 683 (1979)

3. General Features of Hospice Care

Although one of the most prominent aspects of hospice care is its diversity as delivered by different groups, there are common threads that weave through hospice care programs. Certain measures have proved so consistently helpful that they appear to be fundamental to the hospice care approach. It is to these characteristics that we will direct some attention in this chapter. A few of them which require amplification are covered in more detail in subsequent chapters.

Cardinal Principles of Hospice Care

Hospice care strives to be comprehensively effective in every dimension. Because it is palliative care, it is directed at symptoms; however, symptoms are defined in the broadest sense to include not only physical but also emotional, spiritual and social concerns. The interrelationship between the physiological and the psychological is recognized. Just as the objective of hospice care, the relief of all symptoms, is comprehensive, so its techniques are comprehensive in length, breadth and depth. In length it provides continuity of care as the status of the patient's disease changes over time and necessitates various types of care. In breadth hospice care encompasses not just the patient but his family as well. In depth it provides a multidisciplinary team to cope with problems at all levels.

As with all endeavors that are comprehensive, integration of the parts is essential if continuity is to be achieved and fragmentation avoided. Although the various parts of hospice care are here considered separately for purposes of clarity, the communication, coordination and interrelationship between them is essential to the successful implementation of hospice care. The following four items are the cardinal principles of hospice care.

Symptom Control

A key feature of hospice care is that it is directed primarily at sympt)m control rather than at tumor control. This does not mean that there is no place for anti-tumor therapy in such a program but simply that it plays a secondary role in that it is utilized only to the extent that it contributes to symptom control.

The methods employed in control of symptoms in terminally ill patients are the subject of the next chapter. It will be seen that in many respects the techniques employed for control of symptoms in the terminally ill are similar to those employed in other patients, although in some instances there are sharp departures from conventional care. As would be anticipated, there are differences in methods employed by different hospice programs. What is common to all of them, however, is the primary concern with relief of symptoms.

In all medical care attention should be paid to symptom relief, but in most situations in which a choice must be made between symptom control and disease control it is the latter which takes priority. Except for self-limiting diseases for which there are no satisfactory treatments (e.g., the common cold), there are few circumstances other than terminal illness in which attention must be directed predominantly at the relief of symptoms. It is this simple but basic change in approach which so many physicians and others find to be an impediment to good palliative care.

In hospice care symptom control is accomplished with the use of a minimum of diagnostic studies and invasive therapeutic measures. Furthermore, symptoms are considered to include psychosocial problems as well as physical complaints (Schoenberg et al., 1972; Garland, 1978). As a result, hospice patients receive relatively little technological, but a great deal of personal, attention.

Chapter 4 describes techniques that have been used in the relief of physical symptoms. Chapter 5 deals with meeting the psychosocial needs of the patient and family.

As will be noted subsequently, for some patients it is extremely difficult to predict whether anti-tumor therapy in the form of surgery, radiation or chemotherapy will or will not contribute to palliation. As a practical matter, however, this problem arises relatively infrequently; in the instances in which it does occur, the responsible physician must, as in so many other circumstances, make the best possible decision in the face of inadequate information.

Palliative Care in Multiple Settings

For optimal management of terminal illness, the patient must be in the setting most appropriate to his needs at the time and there must be continuity of care as he shifts from one setting to another. Successful hospice care therefore requires a mechanism that will permit a comprehensive approach to the patient whether he is located at home, in the hospital or in an intermediate facility of some type. In other words, hospice care must be deliverable on an inpatient or an outpatient basis in order to meet its full potential.

The most suitable setting for a particular patient at a particular time obviously depends upon a number of factors; these include his physical condition, his home situation and his attitude toward his illness and his family. The input of members of the multidisciplinary team is important in making decisions about where the patient can best receive care.

It has been our experience that most patients and their families prefer to have the patient at home for as much of the terminal illness as possible and wish for the patient to die at home if possible. Although there are exceptions to this preference, the ability to be surrounded by familiar things, the freedom from institutional restrictions and the ready access to family and friends usually makes the home setting a more comfortable environment for the patient. There are obvious economic advantages to having the patient at home.

It is in the provision of hospice care in all possible settings that many hospice programs have encountered difficulty. Programs that can provide home care only may have little influence on care once institutionalization is necessary. Most free-standing hospices with home care programs are handicapped when acute hospital care is necessary. Like most hospital-based programs, the experience of the Church Hospital program has been almost entirely with hospital and home care. Ideally, there should be facilities available for an intermediate level of care in a nursing home arrangement. This is particularly useful for patients who do not have willing and able caregivers in the home or for that small group whose requirements for care are a little more than can be provided in the home but a little less than necessitate hospitalization. We have dealt with this problem by attempting to make our selection of patients in such a way as to take only those who can be managed at home when they do not require acute general hospital care. In addition to excluding a few patients who would otherwise be accepted in the program, this approach has the disadvantage that one cannot always determine in advance which patients will profit from time in an intermediate care facility.

To the extent that hospice care programs are able to provide service in a variety of settings, they make it possible for the patient to enter the program without the need to change his current setting unless there is a medical necessity to do so. In other words, patients can enter the program while hospitalized or enter the program while at home and can, without loss of continuity, shift back and forth between settings as necessary.

In addition to providing hospice services at a variety of levels of care, it is important that hospice care be available 24 hours a day. Problems arise unexpectedly at all hours of the day and night; the capacity for prompt response to the needs of the patient can contribute immensely to palliative care.

Chapter 7 discusses care in the home setting.

The Patient and His Family as the Unit of Care

In hospice care programs, the unit of care is not the patient but the patient and his family. It can be argued that to some extent this should be true of all medical care, but it cannot be denied that it has special importance in the care of the terminally ill. Naturally, the close relatives of the dying patient face problems which can seem insurmountable to them. Some of these are problems relating to the patient's illness; some are problems growing out of their impending loss. Some are practical problems such as financial and living arrangements. Others are psychological problems related to understanding and accepting their altered circumstances in life.

The logical first step in dealing with the patient's family is to identify the family members and gain some insight into their relationships with the patient and with each other. This is not always an easy matter and in actual practice can seldom be done as a first step. Hospice care team members must begin to cope with the family's needs before intrafamily relationships have been clarified. Thus dealing with the family can be extremely demanding.

It should be understood that the term "family" is used here in its very broadest sense. In spite of trends to the contrary in society today, the family is most frequently composed of those immediately related to the patient by blood and marriage: husband, wife, children, parents, etc. Some patients obviously have fragmented families, combined families or extended families. The closest interpersonal relationships of some patients are obviously with individuals who are not related by blood or marriage. Even with the nuclear family it can be difficult sometimes to gain insight into the relationships within the family.

As family members are identified and their relationships with the patient are clarified, efforts are made to provide them with an understanding of the patient's illness and prognosis. This can be more complicated than it seems. Families begin at different levels of understanding and acceptance and within each family there may be significant differences. Preconceptions on the part of family members, intrafamily antagonisms and uncertainty even among hospice personnel regarding the nature of the patient's illness and prognosis can all serve as barriers to understanding of the situation by family members.

As family members gain a comprehension of the nature of the situation, their individual problems and needs begin to crystallize and the hospice care team can start to deal with them appropriately. Necessary practical and psychological support can be provided using the whole arsenal of weapons available to the multidisciplinary hospice care team.

As family understanding and acceptance grows, it becomes possible to use the family as part of the therapeutic team. This capacity to employ family members to provide the patient with physical and emotional assistance has been one of the most gratifying results of our hospice program. The benefit to both the patient and family members which comes from loved ones participating in the care of the patient can be immense.

Hospice care involvement with the family does not end with death. Bereavement follow-up is important. No matter how much anticipatory grief close family members experience before the patient's death, the feelings after death are deep and intense. Furthermore, there is evidence that bereaved individuals tend to themselves be prone to the development of serious illness (Reese and Lutkins, 1967). Much has been learned in recent years about coping with grief and this knowledge can be brought to bear in dealing with families after the patient's death (Parkes, 1980).

A Multidisciplinary Approach

Hospice care is a genuinely multidisciplinary undertaking. Physicians, nurses, clinical nurse practitioners, social workers, physical therapists, chaplains and volunteers are all important components of a hospice care program. Speech therapy, art therapy and music therapy all may have critical roles to play in the care of some terminally ill patients. Symptoms can come from a variety of sources: physical, psychological, social, financial, legal, etc. A team approach is best suited to this situation. As important as is the presence and availability of each of the disciplines, their proper coordination is equally important.

The function of the individual components of the multidisciplinary team and their integration into a functioning unit is dealt with in detail in Chapter 6.

Some Other Basic Considerations

Although a multidisciplinary approach is fundamental to hospice care, to reach its full potential a hospice program must, in the final analysis, be a medical program. The sick and dying patient is at the center of the program's focus and the medical care of the patient cannot be placed on the periphery. From its inception a hospice program must have, not only physician support, but the enthusiastic involvement of physicians. In the operation of the program, physician participation must be available and visible. Physician leadership in day to day care of patients *and* in the administrative management of the program is essential. Physician participants must indeed be prepared to function as team members and to share responsibility. To attempt to operate a hospice care program without active physician involvement either results in failure or the development of a program which exists outside of the conventional care system, leading to further fragmentation and, inevitably, poorer patient care.

In addition to tracing the historical development of hospice programs, Stoddard (1978) and Cohen (1979) review some of the elements of hospice care in various institutions. Lack and Buckingham (1978), Mount (1976b), Saunders (1978) and Walter (1979) provide excellent descriptions of experience with the development of individual hospice programs in various settings. Lamerton

(1973), Rossman (1977), Davidson (1978), Koff (1980) and Hamilton and Reid (1980) and the Maryland Hospital Education Institute (1980) provide reviews of fundamental principles in hospice care.

As a palliative care program develops, all associated with it must be constantly on guard to be certain that potentially curable patients are not deprived of a chance for cure and that incurable patients are not denied a chance of prolonged survival through the use of anti-tumor therapy. In other words, hospice personnel must guard against an over-reaction to the overtreatment which they have sometimes seen terminally ill patients receive. To the extent that there is physician involvement in hospice care, the potential for this over-reaction is diminished. However, even hospice physicians must be careful that in their zeal to provide good palliation they do not become therapeutic nihilists with respect to dealing with the tumor itself. Fear of this reaction has been expressed by responsible observers (Krakoff, 1979; Potter, 1980).

Obviously, the decision whether to direct management toward potential cure or palliation and the decision whether or not to utilize anti-tumor therapy for palliative purposes are ones which clinicians must make all the time, whether or not hospice care is available. In fact, the availability of hospice care probably is helpful in making these decisions. In the first place, it may force the patient's physician to crystallize his thinking, rather than to muddle through in a state of indecision. Unsatisfactory care is the result when those who are responsible fail to make the decision for either cure or palliation clear. In this situation they remain uncertain in their approach to the patient, making it impossible for others involved in the patient's management to know whether or not an effort is being directed at cure. The availability of hospice care can also assist in making these decisions by providing an alternative to futile anti-tumor therapy for those who would like to do something for the patient.

Krakoff (1979) decries "the development of a death and dying cult that is anti-therapy and anti-therapist." One of the important reasons for physician involvement in hospice care is the avoidance of this excess. Good palliative care for the patient for whom there is no hope of cure should be a part of the continuum of the patient's medical care. We must be willing to recognize that we will not be absolutely correct in every decision regarding every patient; however, we must face decisions realistically and make them forthrightly on the basis of the best available evidence. If we create a system in which patients can be shifted back and forth between curative and palliative systems as circumstances change or errors are recognized, we will have contributed immensely to the care of patients with cancer.

It is the author's conviction that it is easier for a hospice program to achieve the integration of curative and palliative care which is optimal in an acute care hospital than in a free-standing unit. The use of a Tumor Board approach is also helpful in troublesome cases. One of the interesting things about our Tumor Board experience is that it has demonstrated the difficulty of decisions regarding curative versus palliative care or the use of anti-tumor therapy for palliation. It has shown that in a number of instances there simply is irreconcilable disagreement between physicians. Nonetheless, we feel that is far better for this type of decision to be made in the context of the availability of hospice care in addition to other forms of therapy.

Another vexing problem in terminal care is the presence of metastasis from an unknown primary tumor (Didolkar et al, 1977). Such metastases may show up in a number of ways, such as a lymph node in the neck, a lesion seen on chest x-ray or a skin nodule. They may or may not be symptomatic. The critical question which arises is of course the amount of time and effort which should be expended in searching for the location of the primary tumor. This is a matter in which several informed opinions and the use of good sense can vastly improve care. Neither a completely defeatist approach nor a relentless and senseless search for the primary tumor is in the patient's best interests. Generally speaking, we feel that a reasonable search should be made for any likely primary tumor treatment of which could contribute materially to palliation in terms of quantity or quality of life. There is no point, however, in exhausting the patient and using valuable time to find a primary tumor for which no treatment will be feasible. Although the attending physician is the one who must make the critical decision, the use of consultations and the knowledge of Tumor Board members can be of enormous assistance in dealing with the troublesome problem of metastasis from an unknown primary tumor. This selective approach requires careful thought in each individual case rather than the rote performance of a standard battery of tests.

As hospices have developed throughout the United States, increasing attention has naturally been directed to the matter of standards and accreditation. This has produced a great deal of controversy and will doubtless continue to do so for some time. There are a number of problems. Few would deny that there is a need for the establishment of standards for the palliative care of the terminally ill. On the other hand, hospices have been characterized by their diversity and this diversity has contributed to their strength. There is still a great deal to be learned about how to organize and operate hospice care programs and about the proper means of caring for the terminally ill. It is only by encouraging innovation and permitting flexibility that this will be possible. But therein lies a dilemma for standard setters and accreditors.

Furthermore, it would be unrealistic to ignore the fact that hospice care lends itself to abuse. All forms of therapy do, but there are perhaps certain features of hospice care which make it particularly prone to such problems. For example, there is the potential for it to become a quasi-medical or cult-like movement. In addition, as hospice care becomes increasingly recognized as beneficial, such services will increasingly be reimbursed by third party payors. As this happens, unless there are reasonably firm standards, it will be possible for profit-seeking but unqualified entrepreneurs to exploit hospice care.

These problems are compounded by the selection of the term "hospice" to designate this system of palliative care. The term is old and has been used in a variety of connections. There does not seem to be any reasonable way in which to stop anyone who wishes to from operating anything from a motel to a brothel and calling it a "hospice."

Finally, there is a jurisdictional controversy with respect to standard setting and accreditation. Two organizations with an interest in this area come immediately to mind; they are the National Hospice Organization (NHO) and the Joint Commission on Accreditation of Hospitals (JCAH). Both are, of course, nongovernmental bodies. It will not be surprising, however, if other agencies, particularly governmental ones, express an interest in having a role in standard setting and accreditation.

The National Hospice Organization is representative of existing hospices and is clearly knowledgeable and responsible. It has developed a set of standards, but at this point adoption of them by an individual institution is purely voluntary. At present, NHO does not possess the mechanics, expertise or experience to survey and accredit hospices. Furthermore, although it serves both free-standing and hospital-based units, its early emphasis has been toward the former; this creates problems with respect to the accreditation of hospital-based units. The JCAH, on the other hand, possess the mechanics for hospital survey and accreditation but has limited expertise in hospice care and none with respect to free-standing hospice units. It would seem that the best prospect for the development of sound and workable standards would be continuing cooperation between NHO and JCAH to develop appropriate standards, survey methods and accreditation mechanisms. It is imperative that standard setting, inspection and certification be cooperative functions of responsible hospice care providers rather than of governmental agencies and professional regulators. So much of what is fine and true and noble in hospice care could be lost in a maze of bureaucracy.

It is important for those developing and operating hospice care programs to remember that competence and compassion are not mutually exclusive. We tend sometimes to think in dichotomies. We envision, on the one hand, the technically efficient superspecialist expert whose affect is sterile and whose heart is cold and who rushes quickly in and out of the patient's room, pausing only long enough to check the easily measurable parameters of the patient's status. We think, on the other hand, of the bumbling, bottom-of-the-class, kindly but inept soul who will spend hours listening and providing sympathy. Dr. Cicely Saunders and Dr. Frank C. Spencer (1979) are among the capable clinicians who remind us (both in their writing and in their work) that excellence does not preclude kindness. What we must demand in hospice care is compassion with no sacrifice of competence.

Although there are limitations to the "power of positive thinking" approach, one of the items which is most needed by a group establishing a hospice care program is a "can do" philosophy. It is a temptation to look at all the impediments and permit negative thinking to prevail. If one begins with a perception of the need, a firm desire to meet that need and a willingness to do what can be done and to compromise on what cannot be done, it is not a complex matter to establish a hospice care program. Most of us associated with Church Hospital do recognize that its tradition of concern makes it a special place. It is a hospital which for years has been recognized locally for the excellent quality of its nursing care. But it is in point of fact not terribly different in most respects from most hospitals of similar size.

As a hospice program develops it is important that it avoid offering more than it can deliver. This is true with respect to the specifics of the program itself and with respect to terminal illness in general. At the outset those responsible for the program must determine its assets and capabilities and deploy these in the wisest possible way. However, they must concomitantly recognize the limitations within which they must function and be realistic and honest in what they offer. No program can make having terminal cancer pleasant, nor can it make death easy for the patient and family. Pictures of smiling and relaxed hospice patients are very real, very honest and a source of much satisfaction to those of us involved in palliative care of the terminally ill. However, they can be deceptive; that deception may result in bitter disappointment which creates serious problems for patients, families and hospice care staff.

Dying children and adolescents present some special considerations. Because Church Hospital does not have a pediatric service and death from malignancy among adolescents is relatively uncommon, we have had no experience with children and very little with adolescents. Most other hospice programs have also had limited experience with these age groups. Martinson (1980) has been a pioneer in the development of programs for the care of the dying child. Because there are relatively few cancer deaths among children and adolescents throughout the United States, most hospice programs can expect to deal with relatively few children. The avenue which seems thus far to have been most productive is the establishment of first rate home care programs similar to that established by Martinson in Minneapolis-St. Paul, Minnesota. Similar programs have been established in Los Angeles and Seattle. A number of hospice programs do include the care of children. It would appear at this point that there is a limited need for inpatient facilities for dying children; most can be cared for at home throughout much of their terminal illness. There is need for the development of new knowledge in the care of dying children and adolescents, for the wider dissemination of existing knowledge in this important matter and for the development of high quality home care programs for terminally ill young people.

Developing hospice programs must be conscious of their interface with the community. Acceptance and support by the community are essential in a number of respects. The preparation of some explanatory printed materials such as brochures can be very helpful. As community recognition develops, some thought should be given to the coordination of public education about the program. This can often best be done by designating a spokesman to whom public inquiries will be directed and who may also take the initiative in dissemination of appropriate information to the public. In addition, he may serve as the interface with other hospice programs.

Admission to the Progam

One of the most important decisions that will be made by a hospice patient is, of course, the decision to enter the program. It must be a joint determination on the part of the physician or physicians responsible for the patient, the patient himself and his family.

Admission Criteria

Each hospice program must establish a set of criteria or guidelines for admission. This is a highly individual matter which obviously involves local philosophic and practical considerations. Criteria for admission to the Church Hospital hospice program are described, and briefly commented upon, in Chapter 2. Before criteria can be established, the program leaders must obviously agree upon the objectives and capabilities of their program. For example, it must be determined whether or not the program will be restricted to patients with malignant or other disease. A decision must be made with respect to geographic area to be covered and other eligibility criteria. For the foreseeable future, the demand for hospice care will exceed the available supply and this fact must be taken into account as criteria are developed.

A life expectancy criterion is a matter to which some attention must be directed, because the way in which this is handled will shape a number of characteristics of the program. Prediction of life expectancy in all terminal illness (as in all circumstances of life) is subject to much inaccuracy and the source of much misunderstanding. As a surgeon, the author has made it a policy to avoid specific predictions of life expectancy for individual patients—a policy which he seldom relaxes.

Nonetheless, in designing a hospice care program, one must determine whether or not one wishes to provide hospice services to long-term patients. If not, the progressive neurological disorders must obviously be excluded. There are advantages and disadvantages to the inclusion of long-term patients in a program. In programs which have accepted such patients, such as the one at St. Christopher's, they are thought to have enriched the experience of other participants. However, their physical and psychosocial needs may be quite different from those of patients with a shorter life expectancy and not all programs are in a position to provide such care. Because the mix of patients will shape the demands upon a program and determine in some measure the facilities required, it is a matter which deserves careful attention in program planning.

The Church Hospital hospice program has been designed for patients with less than a five- or six-month life expectancy. Therefore the referring physician is required to make a broad estimate of the patient's life expectancy. The uncertainties in this are recognized and the physician is not necessarily expected to share his predictions with the patient or the family.

Most patients who are terminally ill from malignant disease and have a life expectancy of more than six months are at a stage at which little care is required. Therefore, entry into the program can be deferred for a time. Conversely, it can, of course, be argued that both patient and family might profit from admission to the program as soon as it is recognized that the patient is incurable. The leaders of each program must decide how to utilize their available facilities.

Patients with an extremely short life expectancy also present a problem. The patient who dies within a day or so of entering the program almost invariably gains little or nothing from participation while using some of the limited resources of the program. Obviously, in some instances there is gain to his family. Nonetheless, we have felt it prudent to take patients with life expectancy of a few days or less only under unusual circumstances.

Admission Procedure

Once admission criteria have been agreed upon, an admission procedure through which these criteria can be implemented must be established. Again, the particular procedure utilized will depend upon local factors and will be highly individual for each program. It may even change as personnel change. In any event, it should aim to be relatively simple and should enable rapid action. Like the criteria, it should be understood by all involved. The admission procedure should insure that all eligible patients who can be satisfactorily handled are admitted and that all patients who do not meet the criteria or for whom the program presently does not have capacity will be excluded.

The difficulties and advantages of making a categorical decision as to whether a particular patient should be provided with only palliative care are described in the preceding section. The procedure employed for making this decision should maximize the chance that the best decision will be made for the patient and his family. Consultation and the use of a binding or non-binding Tumor Board decision can be employed for particularly difficult cases, but they are obviously not necessary in many instances. However, even in the "obvious" case extreme care should be exercised to confirm that the diagnosis is correct; review of patient records, including operative notes, pathology reports and results of diagnostic studies, should be routine. Failure to do this can lead to lethal errors.

In the implementation of the admission procedure, patient and family understanding and acceptance requires the closest attention. In subsequent sections and chapters we will deal in greater detail with the issue of patient and family understanding and what to tell the patient. These are dynamic, ongoing concerns throughout the patient's terminal illness, rather than static one-time propositions. They are also complex issues, highly individual to each case. However, when the patient's physician makes the decision that hospice care would be appropriate, the patient and his family must also understand and agree. This can be a critical time in many respects.

Again this has to be handled on a strictly individual basis. Patients and families come to this momentous personal occasion with widely varying perceptions of the disease the patient has, the options in care and what a hospice is. An infinite number of possible combinations exists. Patient and family may both have a crystal clear comprehension of the nature of the disease and the alternatives in treatment; they may all be familiar, through previous contacts, with the hospice care program. Unfortunately, it is more usual that the family understands something of the disease but knows little about the alternatives of treatment, the patient knows very little about either and both are totally unfamiliar with hospice care.

During the discussions which provide the patient and his family with the understanding necessary to make an informed decision, the issue of initiation or continuation of anti-tumor therapy often arises. Health care professionals sometimes fail to realize that the expectations of the patient and his family regarding prognosis may be vastly different from that of the physician. The impact upon prognosis of certain events which physicians and nurses easily recognize may not be evident to laymen. For example, local recurrence of breast carcinoma and the development of a distant metastasis several months after resection of colonic carcinoma may be viewed very differently by the non-professional and the professional. The professional must remember this, for otherwise he may make incorrect assumptions about his patient's view of his status. Therefore, as a decision is being made with respect to whether or not the patient's disease is incurable, a decision must also be made with respect to when this information is to be shared with the patient and his family.

In each case, the hospice staff members who are charged through the admission procedure with that responsibility must achieve sufficient understanding on the part of the patient and family so that a meaningful choice can be made by them. This requires a combination of knowledge, patience, perseverance, diplomacy and luck. It is expecting too much in most instances to require full insight from the patient and his family at the time of first contact. Nonetheless, a basic or serious misunderstanding at this point can lead to profound difficulties subsequently. Again, individual circumstances dictate what is best in a particular situation, but the patient and his family should in most instances understand that further care will be strictly of a palliative nature. They should be assured that many symptoms, including pain, can be relieved and avoided, but unrealistic promises must not be made.

It is after these matters have been discussed with the patient and his family that they will make the decision for or against entering the program. Every hospice program has encountered a number of patients who are simply not ready to accept strictly palliative care when hospice care is first explained to them; many of these ultimately enter the program.

Most hospice programs do not have a firm proscription against the use of anti-tumor therapy for patients in the program. Such therapy may contribute to symptom relief, prevent the development of symptoms or increase the patient's life expectancy. However, we have tried to avoid accepting patients for whom anti-tumor therapy was still being utilized under the thin guise of these reasons while in reality its sole purpose was to appease the patient's desire for a continued effort at cure. We have felt that generally this was a poor mental setting in which to begin hospice care. Nonetheless, individuality, flexibility and adaptability are trademarks of hospice care and in special circumstances where the anti-tumor therapy was free of significant side effects we have accepted some such patients.

Similar, although slightly different, conditions prevail when the patient wishes to embark upon unapproved or unaccepted therapies. The most widely publicized of such methods is of course Laetrile, although there are innumerable other similar medications and approaches. Not infrequently it is confrontation with hospice staff regarding admission which first makes it totally clear to the patient that he has an incurable tumor. It is therefore not surprising that it is at this point that a number of patients turn to non-medical methods for control of their disease. By and large we have felt that, although understandable, such efforts on the part of the patient reflect a mental set which makes the provision of hospice care impractical. Furthermore, many of these non-medical methods take the patient out of the country for a protracted period of time or involve time-consuming "treatments" which would seriously conflict with hospice care.

Resolution of this matter of patient and family understanding in one way or another brings one to the issue of consent forms for those patients who are accepted and elect to enter the program. This is the legal dimension of patient and family comprehension and acceptance of hospice care. Informed consent for hospice care is subject to all of the uncertainties and disputes which attend its application anywhere. In addition, however, there are things about terminal illness that magnify the problems of such consent. Denial of illness and death, mental impairment by the disease process, the role of the family in hospice care and a number of other factors complicate this already complex issue.

As discussed above, there is uniform agreement that the patient and the family should generally have a clear understanding of the nature of the problem, of what hospice care does and does not offer and of the alternatives to hospice care. Patients should be accepted into the program only after giving their informed consent. Potter (1980) and Brooks (1980), in remarkably similar passages, seem to go beyond what we have designated above as understanding. They draw an analogy with patients entering formal clinical trials. The analogy, of course, does not hold up in all regards.

As a practical matter, it is in the application of the principle of informed consent in specific situations and in the conversion of this informed consent to a written document that the greatest problems exist. Although a major thrust of hospice care is in most instances to foster patient understanding and acceptance of his situation, we must recognize that this may not be possible or desirable at the outset in every instance. There may be patients with a high level of denial who will profit immensely from hospice care. It may not be possible—or kind and wise—to break through that denial in order to obtain informed consent. Patients themselves sometimes benefit most from hospice care if they enter at a stage at which their level of acceptance of their terminal illness is such that they cannot engage in the kind of candid interchange necessary for true informed consent. Furthermore, both the patient and his family benefit from the hospice care program. Should the family of an irrational terminally ill patient be denied the benefits of hospice care because truly informed consent cannot be procured from the patient?

Even more difficult than the issue of being certain in one's own mind that genuinely informed consent has been procured is the matter of whether or not to have the patient sign special forms. It is really impossible to make a definitive and comprehensive comment regarding consent forms for hospice care. So much depends upon location and time, because different areas of the country (to say nothing of the world) take different views of informed consent and because the legal system's handling of informed consent is still evolving.

For what it is worth, a patient entering the Church Hospital hospice care program does not sign any special form for hospice care. He signs forms only in the event that he enters the hospital as an inpatient. In this case, he signs the general consent form signed by all patients being admitted and specific permits for individual diagnostic and therapeutic procedures, of which he of course has very few. To be crudely devious is the antithesis of the hospice philosophy. In keeping with that philosophy, however, we do not feel that it is possible or prudent to reduce the complex, dynamic, highly individual matter of patient and family understanding and acceptance to a signed form.

Patient Management in the Program

Overall Features

In spite of careful admission procedures, an occasional patient whose diagnosis or prognosis is incorrect will be admitted to the program. There are a number of circumstances under which this can occur, but the important point is that the error be recognized so that appropriate steps may be taken promptly. For example, we had a severely debilitated patient with limited comprehension of English who was admitted to the program from another hospital with a clinical and x-ray picture strongly suggestive of advanced incurable bronchogenic carcinoma. To expedite his care he was taken into the program quickly, although we recognized that a histological diagnosis had not been established. Not long after admission, we secured old records from a third hospital which revealed that six years earlier the x-ray picture had been the same and the abnormal x-ray appearance had been demonstrated to be due to vascular abnormality. Further investigation revealed that his debility was related to a severe depressive reaction. He was dropped from the hospice care program and treated appropriately.

True errors with respect to curability have in our experience been extremely unusual. It is rare that a patient thought to be incurable at the time of entry into the program has subsequently been found to have a curable disease. However, it is certainly not beyond the realm of possiblity for advances in anti-tumor therapy to transform a particular patient from incurable to curable. This points up the need for those involved in hospice care to have a mechanism for remaining abreast of other developments in the field of oncology.

Protracted spontaneous or therapeutically induced remissions are not at all uncommon and are one of the factors which make prediction of life expectancy so difficult. They are particularly common, although still relatively unpredictable, with certain forms of tumors such as breast and prostatic cancer and various types of lymphoma. When such periods of remission are symptom-free and prolonged, a patient can be placed on inactive status in the hospice care program, requiring only periodic check and the availability of reactivation when the situation changes.

As has been repeatedly stressed, those who provide hospice care must be adaptable and flexible. While recognizing fundamental standards of excellence and cardinal principles, one must be prepared to adjust to particular circumstances if the unique needs of the individual patient are to be met. Similarly, hospice care programs must be ready to re-evaluate and revise policies as conditions and personnel change. It may also be necessary to attempt to implement change in the community.

As this is being written, the use of mithramycin in the treatment of hypercalcemia is illustrative. At this point it appears that mithramycin shows promise of being very effective in the treatment of hypercalcemia in patients with advanced malignancy; it produces dramatic symptomatic response without serious toxic side effect. In an effective dosage range no monitoring is necessary. However, it is apparently best given intravenously about two times per week. There are a number of terminally ill patients for whom hypercalcemia is a principal source of symptoms. For these patients, the capacity to treat hypercalcemia at home will be an immense advantage. However, up to this time we have not used bolus intravenous medication on an ongoing basis in our home care program, nor have other home care providers. It would be a shame to keep a patient with hypercalcemia hospitalized only for treatment with intravenous mithramycin two times per week or to require semi-weekly clinic visits for this purpose. If mithramycin therapy for hypercalcemia fulfills its promise, changes in policy and procedure which will permit its administration at home will be necessary in order for us to avail ourselves of the full benefits of this development.

In hospice care one must be prepared to meet the various fears, concerns and reactions of the patient and his family. Sometimes fears are expressed, but often they must be sensed by the hospice staff. Most people facing death from cancer are in fear of pain and discomfort. In our society, cancer seems in the minds of many to equal a painful death. Reassurance that pain and discomfort can be minimized is an important early component of hospice care. Most patients and their families have a fear of dying and death. The way in which this is best allayed will depend upon the individual circumstances. The author's experience is similar to that of Lewis Thomas (1974), who writes that agony in the final moments of terminal illness is extremely unusual. He points out that patients seem to be showing us all the time that "dying is not such a bad thing to do after all." This can and should be conveyed to patients and their families.

An often unexpressed fear on the part of the family has to do with contagion and heritability of cancer. One need only recognize the fear of cancer as a communicable disease in order to provide reassurance on this point. The matter of heredity may be a bit more complicated, but it does constitute a part of the care of the family. For certain forms of malignancy, the complete absence of any hereditary tendency can be described with confidence to the family. For other forms, a different approach is necessary. The female members of the family of a patient with breast cancer must, at some point, be told that they have a somewhat increased risk of developing breast cancer. The net effect of this advice must be a heightened alertness on their part without the creation of an overwhelming fear.

The family, like the patient, passes through stages in the course of terminal illness. Among these stages is anger. This may be diffuse and may be directed at the professional caregiver. Recognition of this fact can prevent bruised feelings. In dealing with angry family members, it is usually prudent to explore the causes of the anger. Anger may arise from correctable problems in the patient's situation. As family members pass through various stages explanations and discussions with them should continue. The door must be *kept* open.

In spite of the spectrum of talents provided by a hospice multidisciplinary team, such a team cannot, in and of itself, meet the manifold needs of the terminally ill patient and his family. What the multidisciplinary team does bring to hospice care is ready access to the various community resources available. One resource available in many communities and of particular help to cancer patients and their family is the local chapter of Make Today Count. This is an organization that tries to bring together persons with serious illnesses and their families to help them cope with problems of cancer, death and dying.

It is all too easy to look at the care of the terminally ill as a grim and humorless affair. There are, to be sure, overwhelmingly sad and depressing aspects to it. However, the emphasis of hospice care is indeed upon living. Humor is a vital part of life and terminal care is no exception. The gentle and appropriate use of humor can do things which no other therapy can provide. Its value must not be overlooked.

Patient Understanding

Patient and family understanding of diagnosis and prognosis is an important, complicated and controversial topic. Here we can only touch upon a few practical considerations. The issue of what to tell the terminally ill patient about his diagnosis and prognosis has received a great deal of attention. No matter requires greater individualization than this. Patients vary immensely in the understanding that they bring with them as they enter palliative care and, depending upon a number of factors, they have varying needs for explanation and discussion. Unfortunately, there is no way to be certain that for a particular patient one has selected the best of all possible alternatives.

There is general agreement that in almost all instances the interests of the patient and his family are best served when the patient has some understanding of his disease and prognosis. For the dying patient, however, one confronts the problem of denial; we must recognize that, for some patients at some stages of the pilgrimage, denial is the healthiest possible response. For a few, this may persist until death. To attempt explanations to a patient with a high level of denial is at best frustrating and at worst patently harmful. If *individualization* is the first commandment with respect to "telling patients," the importance of *listening* is the second. Listening is in many ways much more important than telling. It is only by first listening that one can determine what can and should be told. Listening, incidently, is here used in its broadest sense, for the patient sends many non-verbal clues. The fact that the patient does not ask questions does not mean that he has no questions. As we listen carefully, we begin to get the feel of what the patient already understands and what further explanation is prudent. For example, it is very important to distinguish the patient who is vigorously signalling that we must not assault him with information for which he is not ready from the patient who has already come to terms with his prognosis but has inaccurate apprehensions about what lies ahead.

A point frequently overlooked is that both listening and telling often need to take place over a period of time at multiple visits. Patients' needs and capacities for understanding change and evolve so that an ongoing dialogue is essential. In this connection it is also important to recognize that understanding is not consistently a progression; a patient may vary immensely from one day to another in what he is willing to accept and assimilate.

The stages of understanding do not always seem logical to the professional. Very often, patients perceive the fact that their disease is fatal before they possess much understanding of what the terminal illness is likely to entail. Therefore, even a patient who clearly accepts the ultimate prognosis may have significant misunderstanding about what is in store for him. So often the expectation is far worse than the reality, particularly when the patient will be receiving hospice care.

Those who first encounter the patient after he is enrolled in the hospice care program can make certain guesses about a patient's understanding of his disease and prognosis. They are well advised, nonetheless, to listen carefully before they take a particular approach to telling the patient about his disease.

Patients vary in their ability and willingness to relate to and share with different individuals. One of the virtues of the multidisciplinary team is that it provides a number of options to the patient in this respect. It makes available several sources of information about the patient's understanding and acceptance of his disease. It is very important, therefore, for the members of the team to share information.

This then brings us to the question of who should convey to the patient information about his disease and his prognosis. Again flexibility and individualization are necessary, but almost without exception the physician should take the lead both in time and in supervision.

As one begins to tell the patient about his disease and prognosis, several things should be borne in mind. The first is to recall the importance of non-verbal communication. Just as in listening, what is not said may be as important as what is said. Smiles and frowns tell a great deal and inflection of the voice can make all the difference in the world. Secondly, it is important to remember that there are many options in what to tell the patient; silence, blatant lies and stark truth are not the only alternatives.

Mount (1976a) and others have gathered data indicating that most patients want to know their diagnosis and prognosis; the same data indicate that usually this is not what happens. In an excellent article on "Telling Patients," Saunders (1965) calls attention to studies that demonstrate that hospital staffs usually make an effort to keep the patient in ignorance, although the great majority of dying patients are quite aware of their status. She concludes, "These two facts look very disturbing when put together, for the truth from which the patient is being 'protected' is the truth with which he is being forced to live in isolation."

West (1980) has explored in detail the issue of communication with patients and their families, covering such questions as who should tell, what should be told and to whom should it be told. These observations verify what many of us who have dealt frequently with the terminally ill believe. As a general rule, patients are aware of their prognosis even if they have not been "told" it. In most instances, they would welcome and would profit from the opportunity to discuss with their physicians and their loved ones the most important fact of their lives. It has never been clear to the author just who is presumed to be the beneficiary of the cruel deception that tries to deprive the dying patient of a valuable therapeutic weapon.

Although there can be no uniform policy with respect to telling patients about their disease and prognosis, there are some guidelines that can be followed. One must begin by listening and continue to listen carefully. One must individualize on the basis of what is heard. One should be alert, both in listening and in telling, to non-verbal communication. For most patients the truth presented kindly and at an appropriate time in a suitable setting can open channels for making dying a little more comfortable and a little gentler.

Antitumor Therapy

A vexing issue in the handling of hospice patients is the use of anti-tumor therapy. Such therapy, in the form of surgery, radiation, chemotherapy and endocrine manipulation, is employed only in so far as it contributes to palliation. However, even within this framework there are some uncertainties. The likelihood of response of a particular tumor and the severity of the side effects of therapy are often extremely difficult to predict. In addition to the potential side effects of therapy, one must also take into consideration the monitoring which the use of a particular form of anti-tumor therapy may require. The performance of multiple invasive studies in association with such therapy may greatly complicate and even obliterate palliative care. In these matters, one can only solicit the best possible advice and then make what seems to be the most reasonable choice.

Beyond this, however, is the question of balancing the quantity and the quality of life; here the uncertainties of anti-tumor therapy are multiplied by the individual and subjective nature of the assessment of quality of life. It is in dealing with this type of problem that the immense advantage of the possibility of talking frankly with the patient and his family becomes evident. One never knows whether the right choice has been made in giving or withholding anti-tumor therapy in a particular instance, but if the decision was based upon the best possible medical opinion combined with a candid assessment on the part of the patient, based on his own particular values, one has reasonable confidence.

Patient Records

It is important that accurate medical records are kept on each patient. The patient's chart serves the same purposes in hospice care as it does elsewhere; these uses need not be reviewed here. Suffice it to say that the use of a multidisciplinary team makes accurate, clear and succinct record keeping particularly important. Communication is critically important to the successful use of a multidisciplinary team; it is the key to avoiding fragmentation. The medical record is one of the avenues of communication. In this respect, it is particularly important to include entries regarding items such as the emotional needs of the patient and his family and what the patient and his family have been told regarding the disease and prognosis. The system of record keeping and patient charting within a hospice program must be established on the basis of local needs and capacities. In a hospital-based program, the regulations governing record keeping are generally the same as they are for other areas of the hospital, although sometimes a few modifications can be made. Some provision should be made for the coordination of inpatient and outpatient records on each patient. There are a number of ways of accomplishing this.

One of the key functions of the medical record is as an evaluation tool. Hospice care is no exception. Terminal illness does not mean that the quality of a patient's care should not be assessed. In fact, the assessment of some dimensions of care (e.g., meeting emotional needs) is more important than for many other patients. Hospice care should be subjected to the same quality assurance measures as other types of medical care. Such evaluation, incidently, is the key to progressive improvement in the care of the terminally ill. Meaningful research that will enable us to grow and improve must be based on the careful evaluation of what we have done.

Inpatient Care

In a hospital-based hospice program, inpatients are obviously those requiring acute hospital care. There are a number of reasons why the terminally ill patient may require hospitalization. The most common is probably for pain control. As described in Chapter 4, proper adjustment of the patient's pain medication to achieve optimal effect often requires the kind of observation and monitoring that cannot be achieved at home. Intestinal obstruction, respiratory failure, persistent nausea and vomiting, hemorrhage and seizures can sometimes be extremely difficult to control at home; a period of hospitalization may be necessary. Agitation and confusion are also very disruptive in the home environment. In some instances families, either for emotional or physical reasons, are no longer capable of providing care, in which case a period of institutional care may be required. The duration and timing of hospitalization is a highly individual matter in each case. Immediacy of impending death is ordinarily not of itself an indication for admission; a large percentage of patients die at home.

Although the patient is hospitalized because of the need for acute level care, the nature of that care is somewhat different for the hospice patient than for the general medical-surgical patient. Efforts are directed strictly at palliation. Control of symptoms in the broadest definition of that term with the provision of ample attention to the patient's psycho-social needs is the theme of care. Although a great deal of personal attention is provided, little diagnostic or therapeutic technology is employed. No diagnostic studies other than those which will contribute to palliation are carried out; no "routine" admission studies such as complete blood count and urinalysis are done. For all patients entered in the hospice care program, it is understood that cardio-pulmonary resuscitation will not be undertaken. Although "no code" orders on certain categories of patients have posed administrative and legal problems in hospitals, we have encountered no difficulty in this regard for hospice care patients. Once again, individualization is a critical feature of patient management. One can conceive of an incurable but largely asymptomatic young patient with a relatively long life expectancy for whom the institution of cardio-pulmonary resuscitation, if needed, might be warranted.

Standing hospital policies and procedures can and should be relaxed somewhat for hospice patients. Our experience has shown that it is possible to do this without detriment to the care of hospice or other patients. Hospice patients may be permitted visitors around the clock and the visitors may be provided with sleeping facilities. Patient's pets may be permitted to visit. Nursing aides, volunteers and even family can be asked to assist in giving the patient oral medications. This is helpful because the long time it takes some patients to get such medication down can be very frustrating to a nurse who must dispense medications to a number of patients.

The method of handling an inpatient admission to the program depends upon the circumstances of admission. Patients may already be in the hospital when they enter the program or they may enter the program concomitantly with admission to the hospital either from home or in transfer from another hospital. In any event, new patients arriving on a nursing unit providing hospice care should be warmly welcomed by the staff. Volunteers are particularly helpful in this. The hospice physician or clinical nurse practitioner should review the available information from the admission materials.

It has been our practice for the clinical nurse practitioner to meet first with the patient and family and then with the patient alone, obtaining such additional historical information as may seem appropriate; this usually relates to details of symptoms. A complete physical examination is then carried out. Soon after the patient's arrival, he should be seen by the hospice physician. Early in the patient's involvement in the program, usually soon after completion of the physical examination, the clinical nurse practitioner meets with the family alone to review the goals of the program. The family is introduced to the social worker and such other personnel as appropriate. Concomitantly, attention is promptly directed to relief of pain if this is a problem for the patient. Pain relief must come first, before other matters are dealt with.

For patients being *readmitted* to the hospital after a period at home, a similar but abbreviated approach is used. The warm friendly welcome is just as important, as are team conferences to review status and goals.

From the beginning, the clinical nurse practitioner makes it a point to see each patient daily, usually once alone and once with family members. For most inpatients there are daily physician visits.

A few days after the patient has entered the program or the hospital, it is generally worthwhile to set up a semi-formal family conference involving all family members, the clinical nurse practitioner, the social worker, the home care director and such other members of the team as may seem appropriate. At this time problems are reviewed, plans for future care at home or in the hospital are discussed and matters such as funeral arrangements can be addressed.

In all respects individualized, high quality inpatient care should be available to the patient throughout his stay. Except for patients for whom death is imminent and for whom death in the hospital is mandated by circumstances, one of the aims of most inpatient stays for hospice patients is discharge as soon as the need for acute general inpatient care has passed. Planning for this should begin as soon as practical and should be properly coordinated with the home care staff. Not only must there be continuity, but the patient must sense that continuity.

Although Chapter 7 is devoted primarily to a description of the organization and operation of home care, it also addresses some general matters that are equally pertinent to inpatient care. Certain principles of nursing care for the terminally ill are reviewed. Techniques of value in dealing with dying and grief are discussed, as is the handling of the moment of death.

Outpatient Care

For most hospice programs to be feasible and certainly for any hospital-based program to meet its full potential, access to an organized home care service as described in Chapter 7 is essential. Without it, a hospital-based program would be in the position of being able to apply hospice principles only while a patient was hospitalized.

Just as there are a number of options for the organizational structure of hospice care itself, there are a number of options in the provision of home care. Home care services can be obtained under contract with an existing agency such as a visiting nurse association or through public health nurses. On the other hand, a hospice, either free standing or hospital-based, can seek the necessary certification for its own home health department. In either event, knowledge of and commitment to hospice principles by the home care staff is imperative; there must be smooth co-operation between the home care and inpatient staffs.

For a hospital-based program that does not have control of or a working relationship with an intermediate care facility, it is important that all patients being considered for admission to the program undergo home care evaluation. Only those patients for whom home care will be feasible (in terms of location and nature of housing, available caregivers, etc.) or those who clearly will require acute general hospital care for the duration of their lives should be accepted.

Otherwise, the program will repeatedly face the situation of having to abandon a patient's hospice-care service or keep him in an acute care facility when such is really not required for medical purposes.

The use of a day care center (Wilkes et al., 1978) is an imaginative and promising innovation in hospital care. It may enable the patient to be at home in a family situation where the principal caregiver is employed. It also opens options for respite for weary family members.

Some patients will enter home care at the time of admission to the hospice care program, but many will enter home care after an interval as hospice inpatients. In the latter event, it is important for the home care staff to become familiar with the patient at the stage of discharge planning and to coordinate their activities with those of the inpatient staff. As discussed in Chapter 7, the home care staff plays a major role in the provision of bereavement service to the family.

There are certain requirements which must be met before home care is possible for a hospice patient:

1. The mechanisms of symptom control must be such that they can be easily employed at home. For example, although some families are capable of giving hypodermic injections, this is often not feasible in the home situation. In actual practice, the techniques of symptom control utilized in hospice care (as described in Chapter 4) are such that they lend themselves well to home care.

2. There must be at least one caregiver in the home who is able and willing to provide the care necessary. This is usually a family member, although it may be a close friend. The importance of dealing with the patient and his family as the unit of care is evident. It is only after adequate understanding has been achieved that families and friends can provide the type of assistance necessary.

3. A well trained home care staff that includes nurses, aides, physical therapists and volunteers must be available. The frequency with which home care visits by these individuals will be necessary depends upon the individual status of the patient.

4. There must be available in the home suitable equipment and supplies. This may include items such as dressings, oxygen, bedside commode, etc. For the patient who is going from hospital to home, it is imperative that these materials be available in the home before the patient is discharged from the hospital.

5. The final requirement for home care is the ready availability of a higher level of care. The patient and family must know that the patient can be admitted promptly to an inpatient facility if this should be necessary. Simple assurance on this point has made it possible to have many patients begin a successful period of home care when they otherwise would have refused to do so.

Special Considerations in a Hospital-Based Hospice Program

A hospital-based hospice program can take a number of forms. For large hospitals, there are probably material advantages to having a separate unit such as the Palliative Care Unit at the Royal Victoria Hospital in Montreal. For smaller hospitals, particularly those with a relatively high occupancy, it may not be suitable to have a separate unit if the inpatient load fluctuates substantially. Having patients spread througout the hospital in a "scatter bed" arrangement creates a number of problems, not the least of which is the difficulty of successfully educating and training nursing personnel throughout the hospital in hospice care principles in a short period of time. Furthermore, this arrangement dissipates some of the cohesiveness of the hospice care program.

Our experience has been with a "swing bed" arrangement on a single nursing unit; we feel that this model has a number of advantages for the medium size and small hospital. Chapter 8 deals with the details of organization and financing of a hospice program within a hospital. A few remarks here may be helpful.

There seem to be certain advantages which a hospital-based program has over a free-standing program; there are certain additional advantages in the use of a swing bed arrangement on a single nursing unit. Hospital-based programs in general tend to ease the problems of the curative-palliative interface. Transition from one approach to the other is usually relatively smooth in such programs. Anti-tumor therapy for palliative purposes is more convenient in an acute general hospital than it is in a free-standing hospice. Hospitals also can make available to the patient other sophisticated forms of care which can contribute to palliation; these may be somewhat more difficult to procure in a free-standing unit. Naturally, although the hospice patient is not subjected to many tests or treatments, there are times when the easy availability of an x-ray or an intramedullary nail can be most helpful in making a patient comfortable.

The other advantage of a hospital-based unit is in a sense the other side of the same coin. Much of what is generic to hospice care can be of benefit to patients who are not terminally ill. There is the opportunity for hospice principles to influence other types of health care in hospital-based units.

One of the advantages of the free-standing unit has been the presumed inability of hospitals to be sufficiently flexible in implementation of policies to make hospice care workable. Hospitals are seen as cold, impersonal and rigid. Our experience has been that the same hospital is quite capable of providing the highest quality of curative medicine and top flight care for the terminally ill.

The swing bed arrangement on a single nursing unit serves several purposes. It prevents the segregation of terminally ill patients and the related disadvantages of isolation. For example, there are many patients who, at the time they could begin to profit from hospice care, are unwilling to have anything to do with a place which they see as one from which there is no return. Integration of hospice patients minimizes the "death house" stigma. It also provides personnel involved in hospice care with a balance between caring for the terminally ill patient and assisting other patients to reach their maximum health status. This not only facilitates the impact of hospice care on other care, but also minimizes problems of staff stress related to constant exposure to the terminally ill.

It provides far more efficient use of hospital beds by maintaining flexibility according to hospital demand. This may make a swing bed hospice program feasible for a small or medium size hospital when no other arrangement would be workable.

The hospital bed issue is a complex one, subject to a number of misinterpretations. It has sometimes been said that implementation of a hospice care program will fill some of the empty beds in an underutilized hospital. This would obviously be true only if, in the course of undertaking a hospice program, the hospital were bringing in patients who would not otherwise be admitted there. If, on the other hand, a hospital simply provides hospice care to those same terminally ill patients for whom it would otherwise provide conventional care, there will not be any increased bed utilization. Church Hospital, as noted, has a high occupancy rate and therefore designed its program primarily for patients of members of its medical staff, though it does accept a limited number of other patients.

The use of hospice principles and practices, particularly use of the home care facilities, has resulted in terminally ill patients spending less time in the hospital and more time outside of it. Therefore, a hospital that does not reach out to serve a new population through its hospice care program will, in fact, not fill empty beds but will empty full ones. The same line of reasoning, incidentally, can be used to reassure the medical staff in a high occupancy hospital that is fearful of "filling up all those beds with dying patients." The point is that as a hospital designs a hospice care program it must look at its own particular circumstances; it can then tailor the program in accordance with its specific situation and needs.

Clinical Research in Palliative Care

For some of the non-physician hospice staff members—and even for some of the physicians—research may carry unpleasant connotations. It is thought of as experimenting on patients and is presumed to be harmful to all involved. Certainly, no responsible person would recommend using hospice patients for the testing of untried drugs or other treatments. However, if care for the terminally ill is to continue to improve, we must learn from our experience and subject proposed methods of treatment to scientific scrutiny. It was from such study that much of what we know and use today was derived.

Hospice programs will vary in their commitment to research, but all should make clinical investigation of approaches to palliative care possible. Up to this point, the advantages of hospice care over conventional care have been documented in anecdotal fashion. Those of us who are convinced of the superiority of hospice care must be prepared to offer some evidence in the future. Even more important, we must begin to study the relative value of treatments within hospice care. Clinical investigation in palliative care will be arduous and demanding. It will require the development and refinement of measurement tools. Meetings such as the seminar in research methodologies sponsored by the Royal Victoria Hospital in October 1980 have proved encouraging.

Whether or not hospice patients should be permitted to be subjects of clinical studies of promising anti-tumor therapy is another somewhat different matter. Obviously informed consent for involvement is needed from the patient but, even with this, one's initial inclination is to feel that the involvement of hospice patients in such protocols is inappropriate. Generally, such protocols require careful patient monitoring, with frequent diagnostic studies of a type quite incompatible with hospice care. However, individualization and flexibility is again the wisest course. One can conceive of a therapy with inconsequential side effects which shows striking promise for the complete cure or at least protracted remission of a certain type of tumor. It does not seem right to deny a patient the chance for such a response simply because he is in a hospice care program. Although our hospice care committee has been approached on a few occasions about involving our patients in anti-tumor therapy studies, we have not yet encountered one which we have felt possessed the characteristics to warrant recommending participation to our patients.

Financial Considerations in Hospice Care

The administrative aspects of hospice care, including its financing, are examined carefully in Chapter 8. It would be well at this point, however, to take a brief overview of the economics of hospice care.

It is legitimate to first inquire whether hospice care as a principle is sound from a financial standpoint. In other words, what does it cost? For several reasons this is not a simple question. In the first place, the diversity of hospice programs makes it impossible to give a comprehensive answer which will apply to all hospice care. In the second place, hospice care is presently at a stage where very little useful information about costs is available. Furthermore, one must determine the sort of care with which the costs of hospice are to be compared. At present all kinds of non-hospice care are provided to terminally ill patients. This may range from virtually no care at all to extremely expensive intensive care. In order to decide whether or not hospice care offers society an economically attractive option in the management of terminal illness, we must establish which of many alternatives is to serve as the basis of comparison.

Nonetheless, there are certain worthwhile general observations that can be made with respect to the costs of hospice care. It involves a minimal use of high level technology, both with respect to diagnostic tests and therapeutic maneuvers. This, together with the fact that under hospice care satisfactory palliation can often be achieved in the home setting, tends to *lower* the cost of the care of terminal illness. This is true even though there are often substantial costs incurred in providing hospice care at home. On the other hand, hospice care involves a great deal of personal attention and, wherever rendered, this tends to *raise* cost. However, the fact that much of this personal attention can be provided by volunteers tends to diminish the cost increases incident to it. The net effect of all of this would appear to be, at this point, a reduction in the cost of the care of terminal illness when hospice care is introduced in replacement of good conventional care.

The other aspect of hospice care financing is the reimbursement of the provider for the costs incurred. The feasibility and survival of most hospice programs rests on this issue. In the United States at this point the situation can be described as uncertain and changing; it is also inconsistent from one area to another.

When we speak of reimbursement we are of course speaking largely of third party payors, since there are almost no patients who will reimburse the hospice directly for a major share of the care provided. The principal third party payors are the state and federal government and Blue Cross-Blue Shield. In some areas other commercial insurance companies are important sources of reimbursement.

We will focus here on institutional reimbursement. Physician reimbursement, for example through Blue Shield and Medicare Part B, is much the same as it would be for terminal care rendered outside a hospice care program. However, it is pertinent to note that these reimbursement systems do not place a heavy emphasis on a high level of personal attention, but tend to be oriented toward disease treatment and episodic care.

Under present reimbursement formulae, institutions receive no payment for some of the important non-medical services that are a vital ingredient of hospice care. This includes the costs of handling some of the patients' social problems and the provision of bereavement counseling.

Strictly medical services are reimbursable in part. Hospital-based programs are paid for inpatient care in essentially the same fashion as they would be for inpatients receiving non-hospice terminal care. However, for outpatients reimbursement is very limited. Many patients do not have any home care provision in their insurance policy. If they do, there are often numerous restrictions on the terms of this reimbursement. For example, the institution may be reimbursed only if there has been a recent prior hospitalization or only if the patient is homebound; these stipulations are often not met by hospice patients. Furthermore, the amounts paid for hospice home care usually do not reflect the longer and more frequent visits that are necessary for hospice patients. Infrequently there is a restriction upon the number of home visits permitted and this restriction may be unrealistic for hospice care patients.

For the free-standing hospice the reimbursement problem may be even more acute. In some areas such institutions are not recognized as a part of the health care system and therefore are not reimbursed at all.

It can easily be seen that reimbursement for hospice services, or more specifically the lack of adequate reimbursement, poses a threat to the viability of hospice care. The problems in reimbursement are being addressed in a number of different ways in different parts of the country. For example, demonstration and pilot projects sponsored by the federal government, state government and insurance carriers are experimenting with liberalized reimbursement formulae that recognize hospice care and take into account its special requirements.

In approaching the matter of reimbursement we must be realistic. If we are to have reimbursement for hospice care, there must be some form of institutional certification in order to protect the public's interests. This raises some very serious problems. Up to this point demonstration and pilot projects have been confined to a relatively small number of hospice programs that can be identified, characterized and monitored in a way which will not be possible when reimbursement becomes more wide-spread. Therefore, hospice workers are going to have to be ready to accept the application of standards and the implementation of accreditation. It is important that such standards and accreditation permit the maximum flexibility and diversity compatible with safety.

Those of us involved with hospice programs are also going to have to accept the fact that financial resources everywhere are limited. As a consequence, some restrictions are going to have to be placed upon the services that can be reimbursed. Hopefully, an informed consumer public will have some role in determining those services which it wishes to have covered (i.e., for which it wishes to pay) under its various insurance policies.

References

Brooks, T.A.: Legal and Regulatory Issues in Hospice Care. Hosp Med Staff June p. 15, (1980)

Cohen, K.P.: *Hospice: Prescription for Terminal Care.* Germantown, Md., Aspen Press (1979)

Davidson, G.W.: *The Hospice: Development and Administration.* Washington, D.C., Hemisphere Publishing Company (1978)

Didolkar, M.S.; Fanous, N.; Elias, E.G.; Moore, R.H.: Metastatic Carcinomas from Occult Primary Tumors—Study of 254 Patients. Ann Surg, Vol. 186, 625 (1977)

Garland, C.A.: *Psychosocial Care of the Dying Patient.* N.Y., McGraw-Hill, (1978)

Hamilton, M.; Reid, H.: *A Hospice Handbook.* Grand Rapids, Mich., William B. Eerdman Publishing Company (1980)

Koff, T.H.: *Hospice: A Caring Community.* Cambridge, Mass., Winthrop Publishing Company (1980)

Krakoff, I.H.: The Case for Active Treatment in Patients with Advanced Cancer: Not Everyone Needs a Hospice. CA—A Cancer Journal for Clinicians, Vol. 29 (1979)

Lack, S.A.; Buckingham, R.W.: *First American Hospice.* New Haven, Conn., Hospice Inc. (1978)

Lamerton, R.: *Care of the Dying.* London, Priority Press (1973)

Martinson, I.M.: *Dying Children at Home.* International Hospice Conference (1980)

Maryland Hospital Education Institute: *Hospice: Time for Decision.* (1980)

Mount, B.M.: The Problem of Caring for the Dying in a General Hospital; The Palliative Care Unit as a Possible Solution. Can Med Assoc J, Vol. 115, 119 (1976a)

Mount, B.M.: *Palliative Care Service: October 1976 Report.* Montreal, Royal Victoria Hospital/McGill University (1976b)

Parkes, C.M.: Bereavement Counseling: Does It Work? Br Med J, Vol. 281 (1980)

Potter, J.F.: A Challenge for the Hospice Movement. N Engl J Med, Vol. 302, 53 (1980)

Reese, W.E.; Lutkins, S.C.: Mortality of Bereavement. Br Med J, Vol. 4, 13 (1967)

Rossman, P.: *Hospice: Creating New Models of Care for the Terminally Ill.* New York, Association Press (1977)

Saunders, C.M.: Telling Patients. District Nursing (1965)

Saunders, C.M.: *Management of Terminal Disease.* London, Yearbook (1978)

Schoenberg, I.B.; Carr, A.C.; Peretz, D.; Kutscher, A.H.: *Psychosocial Aspects of Terminal Care.* New York, Columbia University Press (1972)

Spencer, F.C.: *Competence and Compassion.* The Gibbon Lecture. Bulletin American College of Surgeons (1979)

Stoddard, S.: *The Hospice Movement.* Briarcliff Manor, N.Y. Stein and Day (1978)

Thomas, L.: *The Lives of a Cell.* New York, Viking Press (1974)

Walter, N.T.: *Hospice Pilot Project Report.* Hayward, Cal., Kaiser-Permanente (1979)

West, T.S.; Kirkham, S.R.: *Communication with Patients and Families.* International Hospice Conference (1980)

Wilkes, E.; Crowther, A.G.O.; Greaves, C.W.K.H.: A Different Kind of Day Hospital—For Patients with Preterminal Cancer and Chronic Disease. Br Med J, Vol. 2, 1053 (1978)

4. Medical Measures in Symptom Control

General Considerations

It is in its attitude toward symptom relief that hospice care differs from other medical care. Relief of symptoms becomes the overriding consideration in treatment; symptoms are defined very broadly to include not only physical but also psychological and social problems.

This chapter is devoted to the handling of physical symptoms by medical means. Chapter 5 deals with the psycho-social aspects of care of both the patient and his family.

The objective of this chapter is not to provide a thorough discussion of each of the symptoms that may occur in a patient terminally ill with malignancy. More comprehensive and detailed consideration can be found in other sources (e.g., Abeloff, 1979), as can information regarding the handling of the symptoms occurring in patients with specific types of tumors (Wilson, 1980). Techniques and experiences with symptom relief in other hospice programs has been well presented (Mount, 1976; Saunders, 1978).

The focus here is upon the treatment of those symptoms which we have seen most frequently in our patients. What follows is designed to provide the guidelines that we have found helpful in managing these symptoms. For some, such as pain, we have been quite gratified by our success. With others, such as weakness, we have been quite frustrated by our results.

Although symptom relief takes a higher priority in the dying patient, the methods employed are in most respects similar to those used for other patients. However, experience in hospice programs has taught that certain modifications in approach to symptom control are appropriate for the terminally ill. In other words, relief of symptoms in terminally ill cancer patients often involves simply the application of conventional therapeutic measures; occasionally, however, it includes the use of unconventional techniques.

Although symptom relief is a continuing obligation of all of the care-givers on the hospice team, the importance of beginning such relief early must be emphasized. This is particularly true of pain. The physically uncomfortable person cannot come to grips with and resolve complex philosophic issues. At the very outset of hospice care, efforts at symptom relief must begin.

Three key points in control of physical symptoms deserve emphasis.

1. Adequate communication with the patient regarding his symptoms is essential. One cannot treat symptoms effectively unless one takes care to elicit detailed information about their presence, severity and nature. This requires both time and a proper attitude on the part of those caring for the patient. All members of the hospice care team should be alert to the presence and nature of the patient's symptoms and should relay information about them to the attending physician. Once symptoms are recognized, treatment must be tailored to the symptoms and to the overall situation of the patient. It should be remembered in this connection that the act of communication itself may be a valuable component of therapy.

2. Careful followup, with adjustment of therapy as needed, is of paramount importance. As therapeutic measures are employed, their effectiveness should be carefully monitored. Ineffective treatments should be discontinued; they add unnecessary costs and, through side effect and interaction, may complicate an already difficult situation. This rule is particularly important in palliative care, where symptoms are the main focus of attention. It is very easy to allow medications and treatments to accumulate; this should be avoided.

3. Psychological and social problems can aggravate physical symptoms. Support in coping with such problems can greatly simplify the management of physical symptoms. Thoughtful listening, simple explanations or a helping hand can often minimize the use of drugs or even be more effective than any pharmacological agent.

The provision of symptom control in the terminally ill can demand the highest degree of excellence in clinical judgment. Careful gathering and evaluation of the available information is often required in reaching decisions about relief of symptoms.

Another critical element in the provision of optimal symptom relief is excellence of nursing care. There is really little that is unique about nursing care in a hospice program. If there is anything that distinguishes the hospice nurse from other nurses, it is simply the degree of reliance upon sound nursing practice for success and satisfaction in the work. Hospice care not only draws upon but requires the finest from the traditions of nursing. Constant attention must be directed to the maintenance of patient comfort. To accomplish this effectively the nurse must be active, not passive. One cannot wait for the patient to complain; one must search out problems and anticipate potential difficulties. One must be alert to special dangers such as the development of decubiti. One must monitor the patient's emotional and psychological needs but never to the exclusion of physical needs. One must be aware of the sick person's need for independence. One must be not only a team member but also a team leader. All aspects of fine nursing care are essential if symptom relief is to be at its maximum.

In meeting the patient's needs, sensitivity is essential. The caregiver brings to the situation of terminal illness some perceptions and assumptions that may not conform to those of the patient. It is the patient's needs, however, which must be met. Bingham (1977) has pointed out that needs perceived by the dying patient and needs perceived by those providing his care may not always conform to one another. All members of the hospice team must therefore be alert for and sensitive to what is troubling the patient and his family.

It is not surprising that there is lack of uniform agreement about methods of symptom relief. For many symptoms, there are a variety of available methods of treatment with no consensus as to which is best. For some symptoms, no therapy has proved consistently effective. Obviously, the clinician must resolve these problems as he decides upon some form of treatment for his patient. Hopefully, as time passes we will, through hospice programs and from other sources, gather the kind of useful data that will permit a more sensible selection of options and through which new and effective forms of therapy can be developed.

Some of the most difficult therapeutic choices in the symptomatic treatment of the terminally ill have to do with whether or not to employ anti-tumor therapy in the form of surgery, radiation, chemotherapy or hormonal manipulation. These problems are related to but separate from those at the interface between curative and palliative treatment. In Chapter 3, we discussed the problem of deciding whether the patient has a reasonable chance of cure. It is on this determination that the decision to enter the patient in the hospice program is based. However, once it has been agreed that anti-tumor therapy no longer offers a prospect of cure, whether anti-tumor therapy will contribute to palliation is still open to question.

A similar problem arises with respect to the use of other relatively aggressive forms of palliative treatment. Invasive measures and operative procedures, although initially quite traumatic, may offer better symptomatic relief than do more conservative forms of therapy. The relative benefits and difficulties associated with such forms of treatment must be carefully weighed. Surgical treatment of pathologic fractures can be most helpful, as can palliative intubation of an obstructed esophagus (Zimmerman and King, 1969). On the other hand, the performance of gastrostomy is of relatively limited value as a palliative maneuver in advanced cancer (King and Zimmerman, 1965). In each case, the decision for or against the use of relatively aggressive forms of treatment must be highly individualized.

This type of decision requires great skill in clinical judgment. Information from a number of sources must be assimilated. The type and extent of the tumor, the nature of symptoms, the likelihood of success, the side effects of therapy, the need for monitoring and a number of other factors must be weighed in each case. Consultation combined with frank and thorough discussion can be invaluable in making decisions about aggressive forms of therapy in the terminally ill. Nonetheless, very often the data about the probability of clinical response may be inadequate.

Another related issue which arises in the symptomatic treatment of the terminally ill is the prevention of symptoms. This might be called *prophylactic palliation*. Coping with existing symptoms can confront the hospice staff with some difficult problems and decisions. However, some thought must also be given to the prophylaxis of potential symptoms, which take a variety of forms and may create some very difficult choices. Should anti-tumor treatment or some other aggressive forms of management be used in an effort to forestall the possible development of symptoms? The use of pulmonary resection as a means of preventing, as well as treating, symptoms in incurable lung cancer has shown some promise (King et al., 1965; Smith, 1963). In certain patients with vertebral metastases manifested only by pain, a case can be made for early myelogram and surgical decompression of the spinal cord before symptoms of neurological deficit develop.

Although the matter of prophylactic palliation is controversial, it cannot be ignored by conscientious physicians responsible for the care of terminally ill patients. At this point there are more questions than answers. However, for each individual patient the hospice physician should stay alert to potential measures which may prevent symptoms. In addition, this is one of those fields in which hospice care programs possess the capacity to provide valuable information through careful study.

Another area in which the hospice physician must often make troublesome choices has to do with the treatment of symptoms themselves as opposed to searching out and treating underlying causes. Certain symptoms, such as nausea and dysphagia, can be due to a variety of causes. Sometimes the cause is evident and the choice of whether to treat it or the symptom is easy. Nausea due to digitalis intoxication is best treated by proper adjustment of the digitalis dosage. The dysphagia resulting from a recurrent tumor and extensive esophagitis following heavy radiation therapy for esophageal carcinoma does not lend itself to treatment of the cause of the symptom. However, sometimes the cause of a symptom may be obscure; in such a case, a decision must be made with respect to the vigor and persistence with which the cause will be sought. In other situations, the cause will be evident, but a great deal of judgment may be required in deciding whether it is more prudent to attempt to remedy the cause or simply to treat the symptom. The patient with a relatively advanced malignancy and the onset of nausea and vomiting due to intestinal obstruction frequently poses such a dilemma. Once again, it would not be productive to establish comprehensive rules for dealing with whether to treat the symptom or its underlying cause in the multiple guises in which this question can arise. Careful assessment of the facts of the individual case, the use of good sense and a willingness to make a decision without totally satisfactory evidence are essential.

Another area in which questions with respect to control of symptoms arise is the subject of intercurrent problems not immediately related to the advanced malignancy. Renal failure, congestive heart failure, pulmonary insufficiency and pneumonia are examples. Obviously, decisions must be made on the basis of particular circumstances in individual cases. Early in the course of terminal illness, appropriate treatment of intercurrent disorders can provide additional quantity and quality to life. On the other hand, to apply aggressive treatment to these problems late in the course of terminal illness may not only subject the patient and family to unnecessary discomfort but may actually deprive the patient of what would have been his most comfortable mode of demise.

The aim of reviewing each of these problem areas has not been to provide ready-made solutions, but rather to alert the hospice worker to the kinds of choices that have to be made. An awareness that others have faced these problems and that there are no definitive answers will, we hope, be of some help.

Specific Symptoms

In the treatment of individual symptoms described below, the dosages noted for medications are those which we employ in the medium-sized, middle-aged terminally ill patient with only moderate debility and wasting. Appropriate adjustments of dosages for other types of patients are required.

Pain

Pain, although not uniformly present in the terminally ill, is an extremely common symptom. Oster (1978) provides some quantitative information about pain in advanced malignancy. Deeply interwoven in the fear of cancer in our society today is fear of pain. Through the studies of Twycross (1974) and others, hospice workers have made basic contributions to better pain control in the terminally ill. Outside of formal hospice programs, relief of pain in such patients has continued to receive careful attention (Shemm, 1980).

For those dying patients who have pain, it must be controlled before other symptoms can be handled effectively. Almost all patients with advanced malignancy fear both uncontrollable pain and the possibility of being so mentally obtunded in the effort to relieve pain that they are rendered subhuman. They must be assured from the beginning, and shown thereafter, that it is possible to be kept pain free and alert throughout much of their terminal illness.

The first step in pain control is to determine the *cause* of the pain. Symptoms originating from sources other than the tumor (e.g., dental caries, constipation, hemorrhoids, etc.) must be dealt with appropriately. If pain is due to the tumor, first consideration should be given to the possibility that anti-tumor therapy in the form of excision, radiation or chemotherapy might be helpful. If these do not offer a reasonable promise of pain relief, other measures must be undertaken. For this, many modalities are available: nerve block, neurosurgical procedures, electrical stimulation, hypnosis, acupuncture and analgesics. It has been our experience that although there are circumstances in which other measures are preferable, for most patients pain can be well controlled with the proper use of analgesics. Because analgesics offer certain advantages over other measures, we have usually selected this approach.

As in all pain relief by pharmacological measures, the mildest agent capable of producing relief should be employed. For some patients aspirin or acetaminophen prove quite satisfactory; for many, codeine-like drugs are needed, while for others morphine derivatives are essential.

There are two important points to remember in alleviation of pain from advanced malignancy; it is easier to prevent than to relieve intense pain and fear of additional pain is an important symptom in the terminally ill. For these reasons, the use of analgesics on an as-needed basis plays little role in the management of chronic pain. Analgesic medication must be given on a regular basis.

Relief from chronic pain can be seen as a spectrum, with uncontrolled pain at one extreme and unconsciousness at the other; in the center there is, with most potent analgesics, an area within which chronic pain is relieved and the patient is alert. The aim of pain treatment is to titrate the dosage regimen so that the patient is in this portion of the spectrum.

For the patient for whom pain has been a serious problem over a period of time it is usually best to begin with the assurance that the pain can be relieved and to provide ample narcotic initially. The first aim should be a good night's sleep.

Oral medication is preferred. Liquid preparations are easier to manage than pills and capsules. Occasionally, severe pain is better relieved by parenteral than by oral analgesics, but for most patients the oral route is effective and much more satisfactory.

Aqueous morphine, which is relatively soluble, serves as an excellent potent analgesic for the patient with severe chronic pain from advanced malignancy. It can be mixed with many vehicles for palatable administration. Treatment with aqueous morphine is initiated at regular 4-hour intervals, selecting a dosage for the particular patient which appears appropriate. The morphine dosage and timing can then be adjusted to bring the patient into that central portion of the pain relief spectrum in which he is pain-free and mentally alert.

The dosage of analgesic required to place the patient in the central portion of the pain relief spectrum is a highly individual matter. As a guideline, we have used the rule that if the patient has been on Percodan without relief, a dosage of 15 mg. of aqueous morphine is a suitable place to begin. Surprisingly large doses of morphine may be necessary to produce pain relief, but as long as they do not produce excessive drowsiness there is no harm in these large doses. The principle of a central portion of the spectrum where the patient is pain-free but alert holds through a very wide dosage range depending upon the severity of the underlying pain. In other words, as increasing pain requires an increased dosage of morphine, there is a concomitant increase in tolerance to the drug so that the new high doses do not reduce the patient's level of alertness. It has been our experience, and that of others, that side effects like drowsiness and depression are in large measure related to the patient's overall condition and nutritional status. In other words, a generally robust patient with severe pain will require substantial doses of morphine to relieve his pain but will, at these doses, remain quite alert. However, the severely debilitated patient is likely to have a much narrower pain-free and alert zone in the central portion of the spectrum.

During this period of titration, very careful observation and questioning of the patient is essential. One needs to be certain that pain is indeed relieved. It is also important to avoid repetitive overdosage and to establish the minimal dose which will keep the patient pain-free. As Potter (1980) has observed, the aim is to have ". . . a patient who is free from pain but who is alert enough to enjoy the benefits of pain free survival." Once the proper dosage and timing of morphine are established, they are likely to remain stable over a protracted period of time until there is some major change in the patient's condition.

Narcotics tend to produce nausea; anxiety potentiates pain. Therefore, the patient may initially be given prochlorperazine (Compazine) syrup (5 mg. every 4 hours) for its anti-emetic and tranquilizing effects. Its dosage and timing can also be adjusted as necessary. Once stability of dosage and timing of morphine and Compazine is achieved, the two medications can be combined.

It should be remembered that constipation is a problem with most potent analgesics. Accordingly, the patient should be given ample stool softener while receiving these drugs. We often routinely give patients on narcotics a senna pod laxative.

Bone pain due to osseous metastases can be intense and resistant to therapy. The addition of a non-steroidal anti-inflammatory agent, aspirin, ibuprofen (Motrin), phenylbutazone or indomethocin is sometimes helpful. Some have found that dexamethasone or prednisone, combined with antacid, are safer and more effective than the non-steroidal anti-inflammatory agents. Corticosteroids are particularly useful when pain is due to nerve compression or to a tumor in a confined space, such as the head or pelvis.

In patients with intractable vomiting or dysphagia so severe as to prevent swallowing even small quantities of liquids, 3-mg. hydromorphine (Dilaudid) suppositories are often effective. If not, parenteral therapy, usually with morphine plus Compazine, must be used.

There are two matters with respect to pain relief in the terminally ill which deserve comment because they have been the source of some misunderstanding and controversy.

The first is Brompton's mixture. This combination of heroin with cocaine, alcohol, chloroform water and flavoring agent was the analgesic agent which many of the first English hospices used for pain relief. Although the substance took its name from Brompton's Chest Hospital in London and was presumably used there for treatment of patients with chest diseases, its name became, in the minds of many, intertwined with the term hospice. The rationale of the mixture was that cocaine and alcohol provided some euphoric effect to potentiate the action of heroin. It is not totally clear what the chloroform water was to contribute; unless the English sense of taste is vastly different from that of Americans, it is hard to imagine that it was to contribute to the palatability of the solution. In any event, various hospice programs made modifications in the composition of Brompton's solution. American hospices had to substitute morphine for heroin. Like others, we made our own modifications at Church Hospital. It is not surprising that as experience has grown, Brompton's mixture largely has been replaced by aqueous morphine or heroin. Single-agent drugs are usually more satisfactory than multiple-agent ones. The euphoric effect of cocaine proved to be somewhat unpredictable and its side effects were disturbing, particularly in older patients. Alcohol, in the volume used, contributed little of therapeutic value. It can be better administered as the liquor of the patient's choice. Like most other hospice programs, we have abandoned the use of Brompton's mixture and find it today of little but historic and sentimental interest.

The other matter is the issue of heroin. It is, of course, available for medical purposes in the United Kingdom but not in the United States. There are those who feel strongly that Americans should be allowed to use it for therapeutic purposes, most particularly for the management of terminal illness. Heroin (diamorphine) is, on a milligram for milligram basis, about 1.5 times as potent as morphine; it is somewhat more soluble and has a questionably greater euphoric effect than morphine. It appears that, for oral use, heroin probably has little advantage over morphine. Aqueous morphine is reasonably soluble and the volume of oral solution for each dose is small with either agent. There are other means of achieving whatever euphoric advantage heroin may have over morphine. Therefore, the effect of a given oral dose of heroin can be achieved by giving one and one-half times as many milligrams of morphine.

It is the author's opinion that two arguments can be made for the legalization of the medical use of heroin in the United States. The first is that, because of its greater solubility, it is more satisfactory for parenteral administration. However, in hospice care parenteral analgesics are employed infrequently. The second has to do with the individual variation of the patient in response to medications.

Patients do indeed differ in their reactions to particular medications; what is helpful and innocuous for one patient may be useless or harmful for another. On these grounds, an argument can be made for having available as many medications as possible. Obviously, these arguments for the availability of heroin must be balanced against whatever increased difficulties in narcotics control would result from such availability.

An interesting observation which we have made, as has been noted by other hospice programs, relates to the matter of drug dependency in the terminally ill patient with pain. From time to time pain in such patients abates for one reason or another, either spontaneously or as a consequence of anti-tumor therapy such as radiation. In contrast to the individual who has become addicted by virtue of drug abuse, the terminal patient on running doses of morphine can often be dropped back to lower doses or completely withdrawn from the drug without serious side effects. We have had a number of patients for whom radiation therapy was selected as the primary means of controlling pain but who had been placed on substantial doses of oral morphine pending the effect of radiation. Once their pain was relieved, their analgesic was reduced or discontinued with ease. The relatively short duration of narcotic administration might explain this phenomenon in these patients; it does not do so for those patients who have experienced spontaneous relief of pain after a long-standing lesion has for some reason burned out its capacity to produce pain.

Systemic and Constitutional Problems

Weakness.   This is a common symptom in patients with advanced malignancy. The first step in treatment is to look for specific causes, such as anemia, hypokalemia and hypercalcemia, and to deal with these appropriately. Encouragement in activity and formal physical therapy can be helpful in combating weakness. A proper balance is necessary between encouraging the patient to move around and nagging.

When such measures fail and weakness is a predominant symptom, the use of corticosteroids (prednisone or dexamethasone) or a testosterone preparation may be helpful. Dexamethasone is usually begun at a dosage of 0.75 mg three times per day; if no effect is achieved, this is increased gradually up to 1.5 mg three times per day. Prednisone is usually started at 5 mg three times per day; if no effect is achieved, this is increased to 10 mg three times per day. As an anabolic steroid, we have used nandrolone decanoate (Deca-Durabolin) at 200 mg intramuscularly each week or fluoxymesterone (Halotestin) at 5 mg three times per day. Undesirable side effects of corticosteroid and testosterone preparations must be watched for. As a practical matter, muscular wasting which could clearly be attributed to corticosteroid usage has not been observed, presumably because the time span has been relatively short. On a few occasions we have used a central nervous system stimulant with good effect for the patient in whom weakness was a predominant symptom. Methylphenidate (Ritalin) at a dosage of 10 mg three times per day has been our choice.

Thirst.   The combination of narcotics, dehydration and mouth breathing often results in a combination of troublesome thirst and dry mouth. For this, careful attention to mouth care, the provision of frequent small sips of fluid and sucking on ice chips can provide remarkable relief. An artificial saliva containing methyl-cellulose and glycerin is prepared in our pharmacy and has been helpful in dealing with thirst and dry mouth.

Hypercalcemia.   Although it is a metabolic disorder rather than a symptom, the management of hypercalcemia deserves some special comment. It is not uncommon in patients with advanced malignancy and it is easy to overlook, particularly in patients who are not subject to frequent laboratory tests. It can produce a wide panorama of symptoms in many different organ systems. Also, successful treatment can be quite elusive.

When hypercalcemia occurs late in the course of terminal illness, within a few days of death from an overwhelming tumor, it is best treated by acceptance as a part of the final constellation of problems. However, when it occurs earlier and there is reason to believe that treatment of it will produce symptomatic relief, it should be dealt with. The usual measures (intravenous fluids including saline, loop diuretics, corticosteroids and phosphates) can be employed. Mithramycin is particularly useful in treating hypercalcemia associated with advanced neoplastic disease. As little as 1 to 2 mg two times per week given intravenously can produce dramatic symptomatic response without serious toxic side effect. It can safely be given for as long as 6 months; no monitoring is necessary. It is usually given as an intravenous bolus with about 250 ml of saline. It is important to be certain that there is no extravasation of solution, because mithramycin is irritating to the tissue.

Hemorrhage.   Bleeding can originate from a number of sources in the terminally ill patient and can range from trivial to exsanguinating. Hemorrhage can occur from the primary tumor whether it is located on the surface of the body or in viscera such as the intestine, urinary tract or bronchus. On the other hand, severe bleeding can occur from non-tumor sources such as a peptic ulcer or erosive gastritis.

Bleeding of a minor nature usually requires no treatment by members of the hospice care team. Team members must, however, remember that even slight bleeding can be an unexpected and frightening experience for the patient and his family. In such circumstances, prompt and effective reassurance can be of inestimable value.

It is when bleeding is more substantial that some critical choices must be made with respect to the patient's treatment. Management of severe hemorrhage involves two basic elements: control of the hemorrhage and maintenance of adequate blood volume. A number of factors must be taken into account; these are the patient's general condition, the extent and distribution of the tumor, intercurrent conditions, the cause and site of bleeding, etc. For patients in good general condition with relatively limited tumor and an evident site of bleeding which can be controlled simply, the decision is obviously an easy one. For already moribund patients with widespread tumor and hemorrhage from an obscure, deeply located source, the choice is also easy. However, between these extremes, the hospice staff may be called upon to decide how vigorously to search for a site of bleeding, how aggressively to look for a coagulation abnormality, whether or not to undertake complex treatments including operations and how much blood should be expended in transfusion. To treat too strenuously may not only be costly but may be counterproductive to true palliation. However, failure to treat adequately may unnecessarily shorten a patient's life.

There are really no useful guidelines that can be articulated to cover the handling of all possible combinations which can occur in difficult cases of hemorrhage. This is a situation where ample consultation can be most helpful. It is also one of those points at which the wishes of the patient and the family must be given special consideration.

Gastrointestinal Symptoms

Anorexia.   Loss of appetite and an unwillingness to eat are common occurrences in the terminally ill. There are a number of possible sources of anorexia in patients with advanced malignancy. A detailed examination of this interesting topic is beyond the scope of this book. What does deserve attention here is the fact that anorexia has varying significance in terminally ill patients. It may be a symptom of hypercalcemia, occurring in a patient with a life expectancy of several months, in which case the metabolic disturbance should be dealt with as described above. Similarly, anorexia due to other correctable causes should be treated appropriately.

If loss of appetite occurs early in the patient's course as a relatively isolated symptom, the consequent acceleration of malnutrition may seriously compromise both the quantity and quality of the patient's remaining life. In such circumstances, it is worthwhile not only to direct efforts at the correction of any underlying problems but to try to encourage, by any means possible, the intake of adequate nutrition. Dietary supplements may be very helpful. Except in the most unusual circumstances, however, elemental diet and intravenous hyperalimentation are best avoided in the terminally ill.

For patients with more advanced tumors and in the later stages of their disease, nutritional replenishment becomes of little importance. Anorexia in this situation is often more distressing to the family than to the patient. As a consequence they exhort the patient to eat and present him with large quantities of nutritious food which often aggravates the anorexia. This is an area in which understanding on the part of the family can be most helpful. They must learn that emphasis should now shift from maintenance of nutritional status to enhancing the patient's comfort through the provision of small appetizing meals. Success in making this transition usually results in considerable relief to the patient and his family. Careful discussion of meal planning with the dietitian can be very helpful. Alcoholic beverages usually stimulate appetite.

A corticosteroid (in the dosage as described for weakness) will for some patients produce improvement in appetite. Tricyclic anti-depressants such as doxepin (Sinequan) (50 mg at bedtime) also increase appetite in some patients. These measures may be tried, but their success varies unpredictably between spectacular and nil.

Dysgneusia. An altered sense of taste is a symptom that occasionally occurs in patients with advanced malignancy. At times one sees a patient whose only symptom is a bad taste in his mouth, which he finds extremely annoying. Naturally, poor oral hygiene, dental caries and other obvious contributing factors should be dealt with. If none of these exist, zinc sulfate in 220-mg capsules three times per day can be tried. Its use has been recommended for dysgneusia; controlled trial has not supported its value. Our results with it have been variable. This is one of a number of symptoms that warrants further investigation of its palliative care, as it can be most distressing to the few patients who experience it.

Dysphagia. For the patient who complains of trouble swallowing, it is important to establish the cause. This may be quite apparent but is sometimes difficult to detect. Most frequently it is due to obstruction in the hypopharynx or esophagus; other causes are not uncommon.

Dysphagia due to pain from radiation-induced esophagitis may respond to oral viscous lidocaine (Xylocaine Viscous). When *Candida esophagitis* is at fault, nystatin suspension (Mycostatin) (600,000 units four times per day) often provides relief.

Aguilar et al. (1979) have reviewed the complex and somewhat specialized deglutition problems that occur in patients with head and neck cancer. Although the emphasis in that report is on rehabilitation to establish nutritional adequacy, some of the relatively sophisticated techniques that they employ are worth study by those who deal with terminally ill head and neck cancer patients.

For most patients with severe dysphagia and very advanced tumors, adequate hydration and nutrition can be maintained by patiently giving small frequent feedings of liquids. For those with a less advanced tumor, more aggressive measures such as the passage of a feeding tube or the insertion of an intraluminal esophageal tube (e.g., Celestin) may be warranted. The use of gastrostomy or intravenous fluids is seldom called for in patients with advanced malignancy, although these measures may be helpful in a few circumstances. In handling dysphagia, there is need for individualization of treatment based upon a careful assessment of the particular situation.

Nausea and Vomiting. These symptoms can be due to the patient's tumor, to various medications including morphine, or to factors unrelated to the patient's advanced malignancy. The underlying cause should be sought out and dealt with appropriately. The liberal use of anti-emetics such as prochlorperazine (Compazine) is usually the most effective measure when the underlying cause cannot be corrected. Compazine syrup is begun in a dosage of 5 mg every 4 hours and is increased up to a level of 25 mg four times per day until nausea and vomiting are satisfactorily relieved. Alternatively, 25-mg Compazine suppositories may be given two or three times per day.

Recently, some reports have been published about the use of delta-9-tetra-hydrocannabinol (THC), a derivative of marijuana, for the treatment of nausea and vomiting in cancer patients undergoing chemotherapy. This agent, which is presently available only for investigational purposes, has shown promise. Nausea and vomiting in the terminally ill are not only common symptoms, but are also extremely troublesome ones; they sometimes can be quite refractory to all presently available forms of treatment. Therefore, the trial of THC, or synthetic analogues, in patients not receiving chemotherapy seems warranted.

Constipation. The combination of inactivity, decreased dietary bulk and the use of narcotics sets the stage for constipation in many terminally ill patients. The use of dioctyl sodium sulfosuccinate (Colace) in dosages of 200 to 600 mg per day plus two to six tablets per day of a senna pod preparation (Senokot) generally keeps the patient free of this distressing symptom. Fecal impaction must be watched for and if it occurs must be dealt with in the conventional fashion.

Diarrhea. When diarrhea occurs, an underlying cause such as medication or fecal impaction should be looked for and treated appropriately. Diphenoxylate with atropine (Lomotil) (2 tablets four times per day) or loperamide (Imodium) (2 mg four times per day) have proven effective in patients with severe diarrhea.

Intestinal Obstruction. Planning suitable treatment for intestinal obstruction in the terminally ill requires individualization. The level and cause of obstruction, the extent of the tumor and the general condition of the patient are all factors to be considered in the selection of appropriate therapy.

For example, when complete distal colonic obstruction occurs in a patient with relatively limited, although incurable, tumor, the performance of colostomy can provide excellent palliation. On the other hand, the patient with partial small bowel obstruction from a widely disseminated intra-peritoneal tumor can often be kept quite comfortable by non-operative means without the use of a nasogastric tube.

For such patients, pain can be controlled with adequate analgesics, as described above. Nausea is generally a much more bothersome symptom to the patient than is vomiting. Therefore, without the use of a nasogastric tube and intravenous fluids, the patient can be given large doses of anti-emetics and stool softeners and be allowed to eat and drink. Under these circumstances, he will largely be free of pain and nausea but will vomit periodically while remaining surprisingly comfortable. One of our patients has described the sensation of vomiting under these circumstances as similar to that of voiding or defecating; it relieves an uncomfortable fullness. Although not an ideal situation, this method allows the patient a more comfortable demise than that which results from the performance of a futile laparotomy at which the peritoneal cavity is found to be seeded with extensive tumor producing multiple points of obstruction (Brown et al., 1977; Osteen et al., 1980).

Ascites. Symptomatic ascites sometimes occurs as a dominant symptom relatively early in the terminal illness. In such cases, aggressive conventional therapy including diuretics and paracentesis can produce considerable palliative effect. For the patient with a reasonably long prognosis, the insertion of a LeVeen shunt can be valuable. Asymptomatic ascites and ascites occurring in the moribund patient do not require therapy.

Respiratory Symptoms

Cough. Treatable causes of troublesome cough should be handled in conventional fashion. For example, postnasal drip should be managed in the usual way and, except for the patient with very advanced tumor, pneumonia should be treated with appropriate antibiotics.

Beyond this, several measures directed at treatment of the cough itself are useful. Adequate humidification of the air using a vaporizer is important. Expectorants such as potassium iodide (SSKI) and guaifenesin (Robitussin) are sometimes helpful if the patient has thick tenacious sputum. Codeine alone and codeine-containing preparations such as terpin hydrate with codeine can be used as cough suppressants; so can the more potent narcotics.

As a consequence of dehydration and mouth breathing, many patients complain of dry scratchy throat as the trigger mechanism for their cough. For them, adequate humidification of the air, the use of viscous lidocaine and a cough suppressant medication can provide some relief. Hard candy and Lifesavers are useful.

Dyspnea. The causes of dyspnea that can be treated by specific therapeutic measures should be dealt with appropriately. Pleural fluid accumulation should be drained, bronchospasm should be relieved with the use of bronchodilators and congestive heart failure should be treated in the conventional fashion. To the extent that such measures do not produce relief, the provision of ample reassurance, careful positioning of the patient, the use of oxygen and the administration of sedatives and narcotics can offer quite satisfactory palliation in many instances. Dexamethasone (in the dosage pattern described under *Weakness* above) has sometimes proved useful, particularly when dyspnea is associated with substantial wheezing.

Congestion. A symptom perhaps slightly different from cough and dyspnea is a deep, moist, noisy respiration associated with a rather ineffectual, nonproductive cough. It usually occurs relatively late in the patient's course and has given rise to the term "death rattle." Although usually not a source of distress to the patient, it can be quite bothersome to his family. We have found that 0.4 mg of scopolamine intramuscularly usually makes the patient sound better.

Hiccups. Hiccups occur occasionally in the patient with advanced malignancy. Although they are frequently due to extensive intra-peritoneal or hepatic metastases, other causes that are treatable, such as gastric dilatation, should be looked for and dealt with appropriately if present. In the absence of such treatable causes, hiccups can be a very refractory symptom. The simple mechanical measures such as re-breathing, carotid pressure and pressure over the eyeballs are seldom beneficial. Amphetamine (10 mg three times per day) is occasionally successful, as is chlorpromazine (Thorazine) (25 mg three times per day), but neither of these has proved consistently effective. Even phrenic nerve block does not uniformly produce relief.

Urinary Tract Symptoms

Symptomatic Urinary Tract Infection. Patients with symptoms of frequency, dysuria, etc., from urinary tract infection should be dealt with in the conventional fashion. This is urine culture and the prompt institution of appropriate antibiotic therapy.

Incontinence.   For the patient with urinary incontinence Foley catheter or "Texas catheter" can be employed in the usual way.

Neurological Symptoms

Depression.   In handling the depression which is so common in dying patients, the provision of *simple* psychological support by members of the hospice care team can often be extremely effective. This, combined with relief of pain and the easing of some of the social and financial burdens, can improve the patient's mood and should be the first steps in the treatment of depression.

The use of tricyclic antidepressants is frequently beneficial; 50 mg of doxepin (Sinequan) at bedtime has been our choice, because amitriptyline (Elavil) sometimes causes hallucinations and agitation. Cocaine (10 mg by mouth three times per day) may be employed for its euphoric effect, but side effects, particularly in elderly patients, can be troublesome. Methylphenidate (Ritalin) in the dosage pattern described for anorexia above has been utilized for short-term depressive reactions with some success. Psychiatric consultation has rarely been necessary in our hospice patients; it has usually been required for a psychiatric condition that antedated the terminal illness.

Insomnia.   Sleeplessness is a common problem in the chronically ill. It can range from a mildly bothersome complaint to a devastating problem. In its severe form, it can contribute to the patient's overall debility; its effect on the family can be the factor that tips the scale to make home care impossible, necessitating hospitalization. In addition, daytime sleeping interferes with psycho-social support and disintegrates family interactions.

For mild insomnia, it is helpful for the patient and his family to understand that loss of sleep is not unexpected and that in its mild form it is not harmful. The availability of activities during the night such as reading, television, painting, etc., can be helpful. For more severe insomnia, tricyclic drugs given at bedtime (as described for depression) can be helpful. Barbiturates and benzodiazapines (Dalmane) sometimes contribute to depression and are best avoided unless other measures fail.

Dementia.   Dementia in the terminally ill patient with advanced malignancy can be due to a number of factors. Treatable causes such as medications or correctable metabolic disturbances should be looked for and dealt with. If hypoxia is felt to play a role, the use of oxygen can be tried; if this does not produce improvement relatively quickly it should be discontinued.

When there is no treatable cause of dementia, attention should be directed primarily to combating restlessness and agitation and at support of the close family members for whom this is a particularly trying symptom. Haloperidol

(Haldol) (0.5 mg three times per day) has been useful on occasion when there is little agitation. When agitation is the predominant problem, chlorpromazine (Thorazine) (25 mg three times per day) can be tried.

Paralysis. Palliative care for local paralysis, paraplegia and quadriplegia must be individualized. The extent of tumor spread and life expectancy are the major determinants with respect to the institution of rehabilitative measures. If there is reason to believe that aggressive physiotherapy will restore function for a time, it should be pursued. However, for most terminally ill patients with paralysis, rehabilitation is not a consideration. In such circumstances, attention should be directed to the provision of comfort and the avoidance of skin breakdown.

An area requiring special attention is the matter of metastatic disease of the vertebral column with or without spinal cord and nerve root compression. Pain and potential, developing and established neurological deficits are all sources of concern in providing palliation. Onofrio (1980) has addressed the interesting and challenging topic of metastatic disease to the spine. The considerations in managing such patients can be rather complex.

Usually, the first evidence of spinal metastasis is bone pain, although occasionally asymptomatic metastases are detected on x-ray. In addition to direct symptomatic treatment of the pain, consideration must be given to the matter of anti-tumor therapy to the metastasis. This can be in the form of radiation, chemotherapy or hormonal manipulation. Furthermore, at this point some thought must be given to the matter of the potential for spinal cord or nerve root involvement. A decision must be made as to whether or not a myelogram should be done in the absence of neurologic findings. In other words, the difficult issue of prophylactic palliation must be faced.

In this connection, in addition to other factors such as extent of tumor, general condition of the patient and life expectancy, the source of the primary tumor must be taken into account. Certain tumors, such as prostatic and breast cancers and multiple myeloma, usually have a longer interval between the onset of back pain and the development of cord compression than do lymphomas or tumors of lung, colonic or renal origin.

Ordinarily, we employ radiation therapy in the treatment of vertebral metastases occurring relatively early in the patient's terminal illness. We have not routinely performed a myelogram, nor even obtained neurosurgical consultation. The latter is usually sought *at the first signs* of neurological deficit. A decision regarding further management is then made jointly between the neurosurgeon and the hospice physician. In those cases in which the potential for spinal cord involvement is high, neurosurgical consultation is sought in the absence of neurologic findings.

Although for the most part we have been satisfied with our approach to the problems of metastatic disease to the spine, we recognize that it is an area that deserves further study.

Skin Problems

Decubitus Ulcers. In the course of the patient's routine daily care, it should be remembered that the terminally ill are particularly susceptible to the development of troublesome decubitus ulcers. Prevention is more effective than cure; the earlier a decubitus ulcer is detected the more satisfactorily it can be handled. Because no totally satisfactory means of handling an established decubitus has been agreed upon and because our thinking with respect to their management is in the same evolutionary stage as that of others, we will make no specific recommendations here regarding decubitus care. We have a routine which has proven relatively successful, but we have no reason to believe that we have found the ultimate answer to this vexing problem. Constant alertness to the potential for development of decubitus ulcers, provision of good nursing care for their prevention, early recognition and prompt institution of the locally favored method of treatment are really all we have to offer. Sometimes an enterostomal therapist can be helpful in managing decubitus ulcers.

Pruritus. For some patients with advanced malignancy, particularly those with unrelieved obstructive jaundice, pruritus can be a maddening symptom. Good general skin care is helpful. Emollient creams and methylated lotions often provide relief. Pharmacological agents with presumed anti-pruritic action, such as trimeprazine (Temaril) (2.5 mg four times per day), can be tried; they may be helpful in a few instances. Sometimes a corticosteroid (as described for weakness) produces some relief.

Fungating Growths, Draining Fistulae and Similar Lesions. Appropriate care is critical to the proper management of the terminally ill patient with a semi-necrotic fungating growth on the body surface, a fistula or a malignant ulceration. An enterostomal therapist may be of assistance.

As with decubitus ulcers, there is no standardized method that is uniformly effective for an ulcerated or fungating mass on the skin. The objectives, of course, are to keep the exposed growth clean, dry and odor-free, while avoiding the development of frank infection and hemorrhage. In accomplishing this we have found hydrogen peroxide solutions and mild oxidizing agents such as dilute Dakin's solution quite helpful. In a good review of this topic, Wood (1980) has suggested the use of acetic acid and some of the agents used for burn therapy, such as mafenide acetate. We have found substances such as silver nitrate and potassium permanganate messy and of little use. If bloody oozing does occur, the topical application of a vasoconstrictor such as Adrenalin or a hemostatic agent such as gelfoam may be helpful.

Consideration must always be given to the role of local or systemic antitumor therapy. Electrocoagulation, cryotherapy, excision, radiotherapy, chemotherapy and hormonal therapy are all approaches that should be considered; a decision should be made on the basis of the individual circumstances in the particular case. On the extremities, excisional therapy may require amputation, which can in some situations be a most rewarding palliative maneuver.

Intestinal, urinary tract and bronchial fistulae can be the source of considerable discomfort and may require imaginative local care. Particularly troublesome are fistulae in the perianal area, which may originate either from the urinary tract or the intestinal tract. In such instances, a choice must be made between local care, which is often quite unsatisfactory, and performance of a urinary or fecal diversion procedure. In this connection we have found Turnbull's (1978) technique of diverting loop colostomy very useful. It permits adequate diversion by a procedure which is of less magnitude than the ordinary diverting colostomy.

References

Abeloff, M.D.: *Complications of Cancer: Diagnosis and Management*. Baltimore, Hopkins University Press (1979)

Aguilar, N.V.; Olson, M.L.; Shedd, D.P.: Rehabilitation of Deglutition Problems in Patients with Head and Neck Cancer. Am J Surg, Vol. 138, 501 (1979)

Bingham, C.A.: *A Study of the Relationship Between Perceived Needs of Dying Patients and the Needs Perceived by the Nurses Providing Care to These Patients*. Masters Thesis Dissertation. Washington, D.C., Catholic University (1977)

Brown, P.W.; Terz, J.J.; Lawrence, W.; Blievernicht, S.W.: Survival after Palliative Surgery for Advanced Intraabdominal Cancer. Am J Surg, Vol. 134, 575 (1977)

King, T.C.; Ramos, A.G.; Zimmerman, J.M.: Surgical Palliation for Lung Cancer. Am J Surg, Vol. 109, 432 (1965)

King, T.C.; Zimmerman, J.M.: Gastrostomies in Patients with Incurable Cancer. Amer. Surg, Vol. 31, 251 (1965)

Mount, B.M.: *Palliative Care Service: October 1976 Report*. Montreal, Royal Victoria Hospital/McGill University (1976)

Onofrio, B.M.: Metastatic Disease to the Spine. Mayo Cl Proc, Vol. 55, 460 (1980)

Osteen, R.T.; Guyton, S.; Steele, G.; Wilson, R.E.: Malignant Intestinal Obstruction. Surgery, Vol. 87, 611 (1980)

Oster, M.W.; Vizel, M.; Turgeon, L.R.: Pain of Terminal Cancer Patients. Arch Intern Med, Vol. 138, 1801 (1978)

Potter, J.F.: A Challenge for the Hospice Movement. N Engl J Med, Vol. 302, 53 (1980)

Saunders, C.M.: *Management of Terminal Disease*. London, Yearbook (1978)

Shemm, D.S.; Logue, G.L.; Maltbie, A.A.; Dugan, S.: Medical Management of Chronic Cancer Pain. JAMA, Vol. 241, 2408 (1979)

Smith, R.A.: Surgery in Treatment of Locally Advanced Lung Carcinoma. Thorax, Vol. 18, 21 (1963)

Turnbull, R.A.: *Diverting Loop Transverse Colostomy*. Current Surgical Techniques, Schering (1978)

Twycross, R.G.: Clinical Experience with Diamorphine in Advanced Malignant Disease. Intern J Clin Pharmacol Ther Toxicol, Vol. 9, 184 (1974)

Wilson, C.B.; Fulton, D.S.; Seager, M.L.: Supportive Management of the Patient with Malignant Brain Tumor. JAMA, Vol. 244, 1249 (1980)

Wood, D.K.: The Draining Malignant Ulceration. JAMA, Vol. 244, 820 (1980)

Zimmerman, J.M.; King, T.C.: Use of the Souttar Tube in the Management of Advanced Esophageal Cancer. Ann Surg, Vol. 169, 867 (1969)

5. Meeting the Psychosocial Needs of the Patient and His Family

THE REVEREND PAUL S. DAWSON

It is beyond the scope of this book to attempt an exhaustive survey of the psychosocial aspect of hospice care and the techniques for dealing with it. Textbooks are available for this purpose (Schoenberg et al. 1972) (Garland, 1978). There is a sense, too, in which such a survey would not be appropriate. The interpersonal relationships that develop in such a program are experienced at an intensely personal level, making it difficult to think in terms of ready-made techniques to draw out of one's satchel for day to day situations. I avoid the "stages" approach because of the linear or horizontal impetus that it implies; it is tempting in a clinical setting to follow such a structured sequence slavishly. A "how to" approach is often impersonal and can generate a false confidence derived from the current mystique of expertise.

Rather, I shall suggest some guidelines that have helped me in my work and have seemed to be helpful to others. The attention here is deliberately personal, subjective (hopefully in an informed way) and humble. Humility is applicable and possible when that to which one relates is regarded with sincerity, with reverence. The patient and/or family are always considered to be unique entities. Each individual is a fresh frontier—a field for discovery, an opportunity for mutual endeavor that is rich in resources for creative understanding. These resources are found not in textbooks or manuals, but in the soil of our common humanity, shared religious faith—a community of genuine concern. Concentration must be deep and intuitive and the climate, sensitive and intimate.

Hospice as Family: Some Considerations
Concerning the Psychosocial Dimension in Hospice Care

Mrs. C., 75 years old, was typical of forgotten people everywhere. Having had no children, she was quite alone in her one-room apartment in a municipal high rise for the elderly when she was found to have cancer of the bowel and bladder.

After surgery, she came under the home care department at our hospital. She lived just one block away. Old, plain, ill, with no friends or family nearby, she was nevertheless a happy person. Occasional dress-up visits downtown were high points in her life; she window shopped, moved with the crowds, fed the pigeons and basked in the warm sunlight. Her health continued to decline; finally, she was admitted to our hospice program. As the limitations imposed by her illness closed in, she became depressed. She began to see herself as others saw her; she was happiest, she said, when she was asleep. Then came hallucinations and confusion. None of us likes to think about the Mrs. C.'s of this world; that is precisely their tragedy. No one cares.

In Mrs. C.'s case, someone did care. In hospice, the number of people who noticed and tried to do something for her increased. She was able to tolerate her situation because she knew that she would receive care that would see her through to the end. One of the hospice nurse interns visited her three times a day during those last days at home to see that she took her medicine regularly; she tended to forget. On her last birthday, the home care staff gave her a fine birthday party. They took her picture; she was definitely a person to be reckoned with. One of the hospice volunteers took her to have her hair done. During the last few weeks of life, in our hospital, the confusion and withdrawal continued, but she was surrounded by her beloved stuffed animals, each given a name. Close to the end she was visited by the nurse intern who had given her medicine at home. Her face broke into a strong smile for the last time. Then this impoverished old lady, with so little to commend her to the world, died as simply as she had lived.

A month or so before, the one relative of Mrs. C. who lived in the city had died. An elderly cousin some distance away was not able to assume any responsibility for Mrs. C.'s burial. There was no one even to claim her body. Then a very significant thing happened. The hospice staff mobilized out of an initial anguished reaction to act on her behalf as a family normally would. The few remaining dollars were used for her cremation. A funeral service was conducted in the hospital chapel; some 10 or 12 hospice staff persons and volunteers were present. Her ashes were buried in a lovely grotto at All Saints' Convent near the city. (The All Saints Sisters of the Poor are an episcopal religious order for women. One of the All Saints' sisters, Sr. Catherine Grace, herself an R.N., worked from the beginning in the effort to form and establish the hospice program at our hospital.) We all knew a great peace as the small box containing Mrs. C.'s ashes was lowered into the tiny neat grave, marked by a simple wooden cross; the sisters at the Convent had prepared the site. Dr. Yukna, our hospice physician, stepped forward and gently covered the grave with fresh earth. One of the nurses had brought a beautiful, hardy chrysanthemum to plant at her grave, but we found that the grave was in a shaded, protected area unsuited for such a plant. At first the suggestion was made that we get another plant that would thrive in the shade. But we agreed that it would be more appropriate to let it remain as it was; nature would provide its own glory in that hallowed, humble place. There was a feeling of profound resolution that we all shared. Mrs. C. would be happy to know how things had worked out. We experienced there a profound intimacy that would never change, that we would never forget. We were all, including Mrs. C., a *family*.

It occurred to me then that hospice is, above all else, best typified as family. The psychosocial dynamic in hospice care is that of a family looking after its own, whether this is said of the staff in relation to the patient, to his family, or of the staff itself. I would like in the next few pages to try to explain what this means.

Family as the Basic Unit of Human Life

Family is an extension of the individuals who comprise it. In turn, the individual continuously receives the projection of the family, for better or worse, which shapes and profoundly affects him. Family has often been described as a microcosm of the community. As such, it is at once laboratory, classroom, oratory, playing field, battleground and sanctuary. It is literally the matrix out of which community life emerges and in relation to which the community's value and viability are tested. Should family life disintegrate, the community is affected specifically. A healthy and loving family is often recognized as a model at the heart of the community—a witness to its own strongest purpose. The Judeo-Christian imagery for the community of faith is drawn from family life and much of its moral sense is directed toward perpetuating healthy and responsible family life. It is through the family dynamic, beginning with the experience of the warm nourishing mother, that the child achieves that most peculiar characteristic of human beings, which is *self* and *other* awareness—the ability to reflect upon oneself and others as distinct entities capable of relationship sharing and mutual endeavor.

Spirit—The Vital Force in All Human Life.   Participation in family life and, by extension, community life promotes the emergence of spiritual awareness and, with it, the sense of abiding significance and purpose. It has been said that "By its very nature spirit is the presence of being, that which first gives rise to history and meaning (Rahner, 1975)."

Presence.   Bernard Tyrell (1975) states: "By losing himself in participation (man) finds himself as a 'presence.' Interacting with other, whether object or person, one is made aware of oneself as a distinct entity." I am here, and I see that in relation to the typewriter beyond and in front of me, and the chair on which I sit. The subject/object polarity can be a trap in which one's own sense of presence exists painfully as an inescapable reminder of isolation and estrangement from others. Our society tends to inhibit the experience of intimacy in which persons are deeply present to one another. The pain of such estrangement can be unbearable; it is a terrible form of suffering.

The communion that can emerge from persons being significantly present to one another is one of the most profoundly moving and meaningful occurrences in human experience. I have seen people transformed almost before my eyes from withdrawn, diseased, tense cripples to persons full of hope, peace and healing power. This has happened particularly in those instances before surgery when persons have opened up and confided dark worries and concerns never revealed to anyone before. In these experiences, the effect is miraculous and often the healing process is dramatically heightened and accelerated.

Perhaps there is no occasion when persons are more present to one another than when they are deeply in love. Henri Nouwen (1974) has said, "to care means first of all to be present to each other." Lovers share in intimacy that seems limitless. Such a relationship is profoundly spiritual. Inevitably, the lovers want to learn all about each other; they want to share history. As the relationship evolves, they want to *make* history together and, out of this mutual endeavor in which lives are shared and intermingled intimately, a profound and sustaining sense of meaning begins to take shape. Such shared meaning is rightly appreciated as one of the highest values in human life.

To be well is to have everything to live for. To possess a sense of well-being is also one of the greatest treasures in human existence. To be recognized as a valuable and appreciated presence in the community enhances and broadens one's personal horizons and permits the active development of personal potential.

History. Nouwen (1972) says, "The emptiness of the past and the future can never be filled with words but only by the presence of man." Time is important in hospice care. Opportunity may be once and for all. Need may require long periods of undivided attention from the staff. The development of themes that arise may require a great deal of effort from a great many people.

While engaged with another, one may not think very much about time, particularly the limits it seems to impose on our ordinary life. Time for most of us is a continuum moving along second by second, hour by hour, day by day. There is the illusion that this duration is open-ended, that time repeats itself. "There's always tomorrow . . . I forgot, but I'll get it the next time around." Our past, particularly the painful, half-forgotten elements of the past, is assimilated slowly, dreamily. Even with the help of a skilled psychotherapist, coming to terms with the difficult areas of one's past takes time. The future seems filled with possibilities, renewed opportunities, "another chance"; the future is entered, also, dreamily and expectantly. The present moment tends to be lost in the progression from the past toward the emerging future. Often we either lean back into the past, "living in the past," or project into the future, our "heads in the clouds.'' Time in hospice care is focussed much more insistently on the present. True, the patient and the family may be absorbed in the past, denying the present or gazing nostalgically at the future, clinging to whatever wisps of hope for extended mortality might be available. But the staff must work always from the present and toward the present. They must ask, ''What bearing does the past have upon the present situation . . . what future can one realistically expect out of the present situation?''

I remember a profound self-observation made by a Trappist priest, Fr. Stephen Usinowicz, who was talking about his own orientation in life. He said, ''I have no past or future,'' and he went on to speak of the ''gift of the presence of the moment.'' Of course, we all have past and future, but when we are absorbed intently in the present moment, with ''presence of the moment,'' past and future are absorbed into the present. The *now* dominates experience as we move solidly planted in its growing edge. It is in the *now* that one finds the essentials for understanding and meaning, because it is in the *now* that one finds the incontrovertible certainty, vivid and tangible, of *life*.

I once visited an elderly Jewish woman who was scheduled for surgery. She was very frightened; I understood why when she revealed to me that she had spent years in a concentration camp in Nazi Germany. All of her family, except for a few of her relatives who were living in the United States at the time, were killed in the camps during the war. I have learned since that such persons are terrified by hospitalization and, particularly, surgery, because the institutional experience is so reminiscent of the imposed controls of the concentration camp. We talked for a moment. My heart went out to her and she responded warmly to my concern. I asked if I could pray with her. I laid my hands on her head, and prayed what I hoped would be an acceptable prayer. When I had finished, she took my hands in hers. Tears streamed down her face. Her eyes, filled with love, held mine; all the compassion of her suffering filled that moment. Slowly, her voice husky and tremulous with feeling, she prayed for me in Hebrew. It was one of the most intimate experiences of my life, in which this foreign Jewish lady and Christian priest were one. Our past and future melded into that moment.

One may find, wondrously, that in a few moments a problem is resolved, a disturbance cleared up, a confession made that would ordinarily take a great deal of time. One can observe in a patient or family the review of a lifetime accomplished redemptively in minutes. Sometimes a few words or a glance or a gesture may say it all. I remember another occasion, when, fresh out of seminary, I was beginning my ministry. Inexperienced and rather timid, particularly where crisis was concerned, I had been regularly visiting a woman in the parish who was a cardiac invalid. We grew close; I really looked forward to my visits with her. I left these visits nourished by her courage, grace and faith. Finally, she was hospitalized with acute congestive heart failure. I visited her there and was appalled to find that she was fighting for every breath, her eyes wild, face contorted, chest heaving. She was a grotesque caricature of the woman I thought I had known so well. As I gazed at her, veiled behind an oxygen tent, I was horrified and paralyzed; there seemed nothing that I could do. She met my gaze, and for a moment her face relaxed, a look of radiant peace came into her eyes, and she smiled as if to say: "It's all right—it's enough for you just to be here." I knew immediately that she was all right in spite of her great suffering. Past and future meshed magnificently in that beautiful smile; the communion we experienced then was its own meaningful history and prayer. From that momentary glance, soon to dissolve again into the chaos of her suffering, we understood all that needed to be known and I left with a strong feeling of peace and confidence in her ability to cope.

Concentration, sensitive listening, openness, caring and commitment all contribute to presence of the moment. Fr. Stephen spoke of it as a gift. I soon realized in seeking his counsel that it was indeed in him an extraordinary gift. But it is a gift that all of us can acquire, at least in some measure, through discipline and practice. It comes through a willingness to share our vitality, freely given without the requirement that it be reciprocated. Regular meditation through which one aims at inner focus and "centering" is a basic prerequisite. This means to be in firm touch with one's own interior or inner core of being. So much of the time we fly off in all directions, our concentration flitting from one surface to another, never settling down, never really consolidating the spiritual resources we all have within us, toward one particular area. "Centering" involves a quieting down inside, a single-mindedness, a clarity of motivation, the cultivation of inner peace. (One description of centering that has been helpful to me is to form an image of oneself rooted solidly to the ground, with concentration and focus of attention being mobilized around this rootedness.)

That can be difficult to achieve or maintain in a clinical setting, but it is not impossible; perhaps it comes down to priorities. There are two ingredients that must come into play once centering has been accomplished; these are compassion and intuition. One must care enough about the other to be truly *present* with him. One must also listen for and respond quickly to clues, cues, themes that may lie almost hidden in the multilayered *presence* of the other, as well as in oneself. Sometimes an expression or phrase from the other will suddenly resonate with something within our own backlog of experience and insight springs into consciousness. Intuition has been described as the apprehension of truth from a minimum of data (Westcott, 1968). For some, intuition is second nature; for others, its use can present serious difficulties (Jung, 1971). But just as one can learn to identify subltle nuances of sound or color or touch when necessity requires (as in hearing loss or blindness), so one can learn to listen more effectively beyond the surface. It is most important to avoid jumping to conclusions or leaping ahead of the person to whom we are relating. To do so is to lose presence. Listening intuitively requires staying with the person to whom one is relating, not jumping ahead or anticipating his thoughts, at least vocally. The intuitive interchange is intimate and profoundly sharing when it is going well. It is a kind of co-pilgrimage in which two or more people walk together, on the same ground, hand in hand, one step at a time. As one seeks to understand, one must ask over and over, "What does this say to me; what does my "gut" tell me?" The intellect comes forward to sift and sort, to make sense of the information perceived.

Memories play an important part in the factor of time with hospice patients and their families. In fact, one's earliest memories provide strong clues as to the underlying philosophy, life style or personality tone which shape one's history. Alfred Adler suggests that earliest memories symbolize one's outlook on life, one's life style, reflecting, perhaps, a dominant inferiority and the mode adopted to compensate for that inferiority, often taking the form of an overcompensation or striving for superiority (Adler, 1969). To use an imaginary illustration, the following early memory might speak for itself in indicating an attitude of life, "I remember when I was 5 or 6 years old, my father, in a rage, beat my mother. I was cowering in the corner, feeling helpless and frightened. Suddenly, he noticed me, and started in my direction. His eyes were cold and murderous. I thought he was going to kill me. My mother grabbed him and kept him from reaching me. I ran out of his reach. I both hated and feared my father." The important thing to remember in looking at such memories is that, although they may or may not be the earliest memory or may or may not be entirely accurate, they reflect upon the general attitude of the person. The object of this exercise is to provide a quick and incisive clue to aid understanding. It should not be used dogmatically to psych out or rigidly categorize.

I have asked for earliest memories of experience with death as an exercise for those who are preparing to work with the dying. This can also be helpful with those close to a dying patient who have a particularly difficult time dealing with death. Sometimes the memory betrays an incident or symbolizes an early experience or attitude that affects the person's reaction and response to death or dying generally. It will most likely reflect, if nothing else, a predominantly negative or positive feeling toward this subject.

The review and recapitulation of the past is seen in dying patients as they try to make sense out of what is happening to them and to discover meaning in a grasp of the whole, the *gestalt,* of what went before. This involves a distillation in which certain themes, incidents and conflicts stand out, interplaying with others and with the present. They establish a kind of skyline which, when transcended, having been absorbed into the fabric of one's life, provides a background for dealing with present developments meaningfully. In this fashion, the patient is able to control what is happening in him.

We are all victimized by our ignorance. Enlightenment, through the discovery of meaning, brings a stronger ability to cope with the immensity of the dying process. Another way of putting it is that much unconscious material comes to the surface for the dying in the form of non-verbal images and symbols, dreams, fantasies and hallucinations. These materials can be brought into the consciousness and understood. Once assimilated into consciousness, feelings of disturbance, anxiety, fear, and perhaps of losing touch with reality disappear to be replaced by an increased strength and greater resiliency. Occasionally, psychiatric intervention is necessary to come to terms with this psychic turbulence. Most usually, sensitive support on the part of the staff or family can provide all that is needed to come through.

Carl Jung has indicated that the human lifespan is like a parabola, beginning in birth and ending in death. In the first ascending half of life, the emphasis is on establishing oneself, accumulating and making a place in the world. The second half, which normally begins in middle age, represents a coming to terms with death, whose approach is intimated in the physical signs of aging, the slowing down that is characteristic of middle and old age. There is an increasing tendency to turn inward in reflection upon the substance of life already apprehended. Direction is toward completion and the achievement of wholeness. In the dying patient, no matter how old or young, the promptings from within urge, too, toward completion, rounding out, wholeness. This is as true in the young as in those who are dying at the end of a normal lifespan.

Jung's concept of the *shadow* figures significantly in that descending portion of life. When one goes with the whole-making process at that stage, he enters into what Jung called individuation, the articulation of the individuality that characterizes a human life. The *shadow* is an unconscious reservoir of undeveloped, neglected, rejected elements in the psychic makeup of each person. There is a dark, threatening, rough, even evil character to this shadow, which is often represented in dreams by a person who threatens to hurt or kill the dreamer. Jung points out that the shadow contains psychic energy which, although repressed or suppressed, does not go away; because it is not channeled it festers and rankles seeking an outlet. If there is no room for the shadow to be expressed in one's conscious life, it becomes truly dangerous; it seeps through the cracks, finding expression in hidden, unexpected, destructive ways. Because it is unconscious, the *shadow* can only be detected in dreams, phantasies and projections. As Whitmont (1969) has pointed out, we can get a glimpse of our shadow, in the mirror as it were, by noting the type of person we instinctively dislike for no good cause or reason. In fact, when we meet someone who resonates with our own *shadow,* it is projected onto that person so that our dislike is a reflection of the repellent character of our own shadow. Jung indicated that the *shadow* plays an active part in a healthy attempt (individuation) to come to terms with the requirements of the second half of life. In order to be whole, there is need to become acquainted with the *shadow,* (always carefully, as with a volatile and somewhat unpredictable roughneck), and even to assimilate some of its characteristics into our personality. We may end up being less neat but will certainly be more human. (There but for the grace of God go I.) In the dying person, there is an increasing need to come to terms with and assimilate the darker, less developed side of his nature, which is brought to the fore in part because he is progressively becoming in an unavoidable way less attractive, weaker and less independent. In working closely with such people, one sometimes finds his shadow projected onto oneself. A creative response rather than a defensive reaction is indicated when this happens. Carrying another's projection, although painful, can help to clarify the issues as long as one understands what is happening and listens so as to read the underlying message. I recall a visit to a patient who was about to go to surgery. As I entered the room, a stranger to this man, he turned to me in fury, eyes blazing, his face livid. I asked, "Why are you so angry?" He suddenly stopped and explained in desperation that he had just come into the hospital; he was due to go to surgery in a few hours and no one had talked to him about his coming operation. For all he knew, he would go to the operating room without anyone knowing who he was; could he even be sure that they would do the right surgery on him? He felt anonymous, cheated and unrecognized. I listened to him and left immediately to talk to the head nurse on the floor. In a few minutes she came with me, sat down beside him and explained exactly what to expect. He responded calmly and quietly. When I had first entered his room, I came not as a clinical person, but as a fellow human being, vulnerable and non-clinical as he was. I received his projection and was able, through listening at a deeper level, to go past his hostile affront to hear his anxiety and fear and was thereby able to help him better to understand his situation.

We, the staff, sometimes project our *shadow* onto the patient, his family or even fellow staff members. When we are faced, in the other, with someone we unreasonably dislike or resist, we can assume that the *shadow,* our *shadow,* is in the picture. We must ask, "Is there anything in me that I see in the person before me; am I seeing that person as he/she really is, or am I looking at my own *shadow* image?" It is not easy to be clear about this, but the exercise of careful and honest assessment can help clear the air and the experience of meeting and dealing creatively with our own shadow in others can be a growth experience for us.

Agnes Sanford (1947) presents an excellent exercise for healing the emotions or memories that, because they are painful or unresolved, poison and plague us, even though half forgotten. She presents this in the context of confession and forgiveness before God, but it can also be used as I suggest here. Relax with pencil and paper at hand. Divide your life into seven periods. Dealing with each period separately, try to remember any unresolved or uncomfortable memories from that time span. Write them down simply and quickly; after the list is completed put it aside. Allowing some time to elapse, go on to the next period and continue in like fashion on through the seven periods. Once this list is completed one can deal with the significantly difficult and painful memories by using a device suggested by Dennis and Matthew Lynn (1978), which is based on the five stages of dying enumerated by Elizabeth Kubler-Ross. These are denial—I don't admit I was ever hurt; anger—I blame others for hurting and destroying me; bargaining—I set up conditions to be fulfilled before I'm ready to forgive;

depression—I blame myself for letting hurt destroy me; acceptance—I look forward to growth from hurt. Applying these stages to the significant memories listed helps to bring them into perspective, and bring those persons involved in the memories into clear focus. It can set us up for forgiveness, healing and reconciliation. This exercise can be a useful tool for those patients and family members who are dealing with painful memories and particularly for those patients who are embarked on the recapitulation process.

Meaning. Existence without meaning becomes intolerable. Viktor Frankl (1963) has pointed out that when life is deprived of meaning, spontaneous death often follows. Such deprivation leads to death of the spirit and life simply ceases.

Perhaps this is what we dread most as we contemplate death or dying; the extinction of meaning, all the more terrible should awareness remain. There is, then, literally nothing to live for.

We all long for a time and place when our spirits have found a home, where history and meaning are shared deeply and where the members of the fellowship in which such sharing takes place are deeply present to one another in love. Much of the appeal of the Church as God's family stems from such longing. Heaven, as a condition of heightened existence free of conflict and mortality in which one is present with loved ones, resonates with that same longing. To be at home in the universe, free of the limits of time and space, in a climate of love and peace is integral with the deeper spiritual experiences that mark every human life. I'm speaking of those moments when time is forgotten, is in a sense unimportant, when the limits of our existence as mortals seem to fall away and one's own existence is experienced as of a piece with all that is.

The Hebrew word *Shalom* comes to mind. Amongst the rich meanings of this word is completeness, in the sense of rounding something out, finishing an ongoing process less understood as an objective gained than as the achievement of wholeness and completeness. There is also a social sense of the word. It is often used as a term of greeting in a social setting, as if to say, "May you and I participate in wholeness and the kind of completion that bespeaks not just harmony and the cessation of strife, but brotherhood—a family unit." The word suggests a unity in diversity, the lion and the lamb lying down together and the sword recast into a plow blade that can be used together for our mutual benefit. The word is used many times in the Bible. It announced the birth of Christ; it was used by the angels as they addressed the shepherds in the fields. It was used by Christ with his disciples after his crucifixion in the resurrection appearances. Here it resonates with the terrible event just past and at the same time opens out into the future. Peace, that awesome serenity, holy and powerful, sometimes can be seen in persons close to death. It is peace in the midst of, and achieved through, great suffering. Its power is all the more impressive because there is well-being in it, a kind of victory in spite of all hell. To be able to die well is to make a magnificent witness to the indestructability of the human spirit. It is a great hymn of hope and victory to those of us who look often into the face of death.

Clearly, history and meaning do find their source in that presence of being that is spirit, realized in individual and communal life. Being well means being complete and whole and being fully alive.

In dealing with dying persons, it is important not to confuse being cured with being well. In terminal illness, cure may be out of the question. However, paradoxically, one can be increasingly well as death draws near. Some of the most powerfully healthy persons I have known have been so immediately before death. Their *presence of being* seems to extend beyond the limits of mortality. This is not to imply that they have achieved a *perfection* of being; it is rather a *completeness* of being at that particular moment. One might wish to say, "This person is completely whole, even though it is clear that there is much left for him to accomplish were he to live." Michael K. Bice (1978), in a fascinating article titled "The Healing of the Dying," quotes Erik Erikson who, speaking about the final stage of ego development, says, "it is the acceptance of one's one and only life cycle as something that had to be and that, by necessity, permitted of no substitutions. . . In such final consolidation, death loses its sting." Bice goes on to quote a doctor whose patient had died well, close to her family, "What was not lost was an intact person, and, it is to be hoped, an intact and functioning bereaved family." Bice comments: "That is true wholeness. That is dying healthy."

Family Matters.   The goal in good hospice care is to provide excellent clinical palliative care and to promote well-being in the patient and in the family. Family here refers not just to the family of the patient. As emphasized by the discussion above, *family* refers to the milieu generated by and within the hospice staff as well. Sometimes this means simply that the hospice staff assumes the role of surrogate family, but it can and should mean too that the staff functions in its own right as a family, a kind of model witnessing to and enabling healthy family life as a matter of principle and *raison d'être*. Should this family sense be jeopardized, the staff suffers and disintegrates; the program loses its meaning and itself dies spiritually, however disciplined and effective it may be clinically.

The level of concentration and intensity in hospice work is unusually high. People who work in such programs are subject to all the stresses, burn-outs and depressions that have come to be recognized as a chronic threat to those engaged in the helping professions. Breakdown has much less to do with the spectre of death hovering over such work than with emotional and spiritual depletion. Depletion can be controlled so long as we function as part of a larger whole. The drain on one person working alone can be exhausting. When the investment of energy is shared with other members of the staff so that the burden is lessened, the depletion factor is not quite so significant. The nourishment received from the hospice *family* provides a resource that makes the difference between burnout and a good work-out. Admitting the family, the volunteers and the patient himself into this community of concern and mutual support means that no one person is left alone; no one person is drained dry.

One must act upon opportunities as they occur; there rarely is another. An unexpected crisis or pressures related to private life can be the straw that breaks the camel's back. In our experience, the staff instinctively rallies like a family in response to trouble with one of its members. The sensitivity, the caring and the nurturing attention that characterizes the staff's attitude toward patients and their families are then directed toward the trouble spot. The results are extraordinarily positive. Those on the staff especially skilled in counseling make themselves available. At such times, the teamwork that is so vital a part of any hospice program is revealed in its deeper, family-like dimensions.

Mrs. H., the bearer of a European title, was a woman of vivid and parlous achievement. Beautiful and exciting in her youth, she lived life to the brim. Married several times, she sometimes left the children of each marriage with extended family as she undertook new adventures. She was much chastened when she came into our hospice program. Having lost her beauty, her youthful vitality and her fortune, she was dependent upon her children and her last husband for spiritual and sometimes financial support. Her disease was such that she was faced with the real possibility of a catastrophic hemorrhage or closure of the throat. She begged to be able to die in the hospital; it was learned that she feared that she would hemorrhage or choke at home without the necessary clinical resources to help her. All of her children but one were alienated for one reason or another from her and from one another. The hospice staff decided to try to call them all together in hopes that their differences might be put aside so that they could support their mother. The prospects for success were not good. To our surprise all of the children with their mates were present for the meeting, ostensibly to discuss the mother's condition. Suddenly, they began talking to one another, listening to one another; they began to function as a family. A schedule was established to enable them to take turns being with their mother around the clock until her death. She was able to let go and found a strong measure of peace as her family rallied at her side. One son who had been particularly estranged leaned close to his mother at one of his visits, kissed her, and said, ''Mother, I love you.'' Her face beaming, she said to one of the staff, ''I never thought I would hear those words from him ever again.'' The family learned to communicate, to relate together again as a *family,* perhaps more intimately than had ever been the case before. Mrs. H. died, as she wished, in the hospital, in peace, with her family at her side.

Elsewhere, I have referred to guilt as the failure (or estimation of failure) of love and/or responsibility (Hamilton and Reid, 1980). Guilt thwarts the very process that will heal it, which is reconciliation and restitution. In so far as injustice was involved in this failure, anger (as the reaction to injustice) fuels guilt as it veils the shame that makes an encounter with the offended party so difficult. Nowhere is this more vividly exemplified than when a patient or family experiencing the loss of a loved one becomes alienated from God. "Why does God allow this to happen? Why am I/are we being punished? Why has God abandoned us?" Anger wells up against God. Behind this anger, one often finds old guilt from past failures of love and responsibility toward God. This guilt is heightened as the anger toward God increases.

One must regard this as a family problem. This is clear when one acknowledges the many references to the Fatherhood of God in Holy Scripture. If God is as a father (in the most familiar sense, Abba, as Christ would have us believe) to us, then in his infinite wisdom and love he must be a *consummate* father to us whom he regards as members of his own family. Surely he must be able to understand our anger at such a time. Indeed, as an exceptional father he will help us toward restoration of a healthier relationship—a reconciliation based on fresh understanding, a new level of maturity and loving support of our own best interests.

Anger is dissipated most effectively by working toward restitution of the injustice, or perceived injustice, that precipitated it. Guilt dissolves when reconciliation occurs with the loved one, when loving communication is restored and mutual responsibility for the terms of the relationship is again assumed.

This, however, does not eliminate the problem of suffering. Cicely Saunders has pointed out the many faces of suffering; it has not only a physical characteristic, but social, spiritual, emotional and mental significance as well. There is no area of human experience that is more difficult to understand, that so mysteriously eludes management. Suffering can only be understood in relation to human freedom, the catapult to awareness and the ability to transcend that distinguishes human beings. Humans have the capacity to select from alternatives, to make choices and to contemplate the ramifications of those choices, to discriminate and judge. The effects of wrong or counterproductive choices, as well as the happier type, are imprinted upon our character, our personality, our destiny, our community. When one speculates upon the age of human civilization, the implications of human choice become staggering. Just as an individual is shaped, scarred and perhaps even crippled by the poor choices and stretched, ennobled and fulfilled by the positive choices he makes throughout a normal lifespan, so we can begin to appreciate the cumulative effect on humankind of the myriad decisions of its members throughout history. In exercising our freedom, we have, along with elements from our own field of possibilities and limitations (genetic equipment, cultural conditioning, etc.) to consider also that of our race, the background of human history, our own social circumstances, etc. Should we try to take all of this into account whenever a significant decision has to be made, we would be paralyzed. All too often we are faced with a choice between alternatives neither of which is preferable. We live with our own mistakes and those of our race. We are all victimized by the mistakes others have made.

Inevitably God receives the blame for much human suffering that "does not make sense.'' If he is a just and loving God, how can he tolerate the pain and the injustice about which we are speaking? Perhaps we cannot find happy answers to that question, particularly if we ask the question out of our own great suffering. But if, indeed, we are free agents within the obvious limits of our animal mortality and if our creator respects that freedom primarily as a necessary condition for loving response, then he cannot continuously rescue us from painful or tragic situations without reneging on our human freedom. A *deus ex machina*[1] may be appropriate for robots, the existences of which are completely determined, but not for free agents. If God is love and he seeks to love and wishes to be loved by the one segment of his creation that is capable of intelligent relationship, then he will try every means available to heal and save his broken and spoiled creation within the terms of freedom and shared responsibility. For Christians, the wonder of Christ is that he opened a way to God from within human history in such a way that human freedom is not compromised or circumscribed, but brought into its most creative possibilities for sound human evolution.

In conclusion, just as a model human father has the capacity for great wisdom, patience, forbearance and loving concern for his children, never really giving up on them, so no less and much more must be expected of the heavenly Father. The author of the 23rd Psalm understood this supremely well.

Summary

If we are to be of help to those who suffer, we must first be present with them. This is impossible unless we allow our own pain and suffering to resonate to some degree with theirs. ''I am where you are, and I know what it is like.'' It must be admitted that what the other is experiencing is unique; that must be respected. But there is a surprising resource of human affinity, much of it programmed into our racial memory. Our intuitive powers enable us to empathize through imagination; this helps when the sufferer begins to know that we *want* to understand, to share the burden of suffering. There is no room in such sharing for maudlin sentimentality.

I'm reminded of John Macquarrie's (1966) explication of the Christian conception of love: *agape*. He calls it ''letting-be,'' in two senses of the word. These are respecting the privacy and independence of the other, granting him the prerogative to be his own unique self, and at the same time enabling him to be, pulling for him and for his well-being.

---

[1] A device used in Greek drama whereby a deity would appear to resolve a complicated or impossible situation. The actor impersonating the deity would appear above the other actors, sometimes descending into the scene by the use of a mechanical apparatus.

Sharing history is important in maintaining presence. Opening one's life experience, one's life story to another requires trust and a kind of open intimacy that is typical of sound family interrelationship. Meaning is spun out of this kind of trusting fellowing or profound meeting, which, if motivated by caring love ("letting-be"), brings out the best in the other.

Martin Buber (1965) speaks to this communion, one with another, "Man exists anthropologically not in his isolation, but in the completeness of the relation between man and man; what humanity *is* can be properly grasped only in vital reciprocity." He goes on to say, "The dynamic glory of the being of man is first bodily present in the relation between two men each of whom in meaning the other also means the highest to which this person is called, and serves the self-realization of this human life as one true to creation without wishing to impose on the other anything of his own realization." In a healthy family, the members know when to let go of one another so as to foster independence and growth. This can be painful. It can mean terminating a mutually nourishing relationship. It can mean taking the risk that the other can make it on his own and *needs* to make it on his own. It can mean being displaced, not being needed any longer. I remember a situation in which I had spent several months relating well to a woman who, as she approached death, was depressed and withdrawn. I had been able to bring her the sacraments and we had long significant talks together. Overall, her response was dramatic. She regained her sense of well-being as death drew near. I had met her family only fleetingly. At the last, I was called late in the evening and was asked to visit her at the hospital. The family was there; there were her husband, two sons, and a niece (who was an employee of the hospital). She was semi-comatose and sinking quickly. I was sure she would not make it through the night. The family clearly appreciated my visit. I had come to feel very close to this lady and was prepared to wait at her bedside with the family through the night. After an hour or so, I was approached by the niece who explained that the family was all right now and I needn't stay. My reaction was a mixture of hurt at being "dismissed" and impatience with myself that I had not read the situation and left earlier. Upon reflection, I came to see that this was much less complicated than I was making it. The patient to whom I had become attached was all right; the support that I had given right after my arrival was all that was required. The family needed to be alone together. The niece's approach was a correct and appropriate one; she did not feel that she had to play games with me, and she felt free to be honest. This is how it is in a sound family. We can be honest with one another and speak simply and directly without fear of being misunderstood. If we appreciate this point, we begin to learn the limits of our involvement and the degree to which we can contribute creatively in a given situation. Knowing how to "finish" is a fine and necessary art to be cultivated by hospice staff, as in any family where some may be less needed than others at a particular time.

There is a temptation in hospice work to feel that nothing less than resolution and/or meaningfulness is acceptable. Some patients and families pass through our program without evidencing an extraordinary need beyond the caring, clinically competent attention that is basic for hospice care. Others come to the close of our experience with them as problematical as when they began. This may reflect on the inadequacy of our skills, but it may also stem from a condition that is normal for that particular family. The most we can do in such an instance is to be available in an open-ended way.

Families are torn and crippled by the loss of a loved one, whether the climate in that family has always been cohesive and close or not. As the patient dies, it is as though an essential part of the family organism dies as well. It can seem as though life is impossible for the future. A great abyss, empty and frightening, is left in the family and the lives of the individual members. Where staff is intensely involved with the patient and family, they are affected as well. This is the cost of investing ourselves in the lives of others. In spite of this devastation, normally, the total person begins to respond to such loss in a creative and unexpected way. Eventually growth occurs that might not have been possible except for the loss experienced. We are never previously aware of our inner capacity for growth and adaptation or our potential for creative response in the face of a dreaded threat to our equilibrium. One is never the same after such a loss, but we find in retrospect that there are compensations. New possibilities present themselves for the sound completion of our lives, our destinies. Communal or family support is necessary if we are to respond to the challenge they represent.

It is typical of such a time that everything appears to be different and strange. There is a "florescence" which at first is frightening and confusing in its promise of new directions and possibilities. Gradually, signposts emerge from that sea of new frontiers and the configuration for a new way commands attention, often urgently. In a real sense, all that opens out afresh comes from the soil of the relationships that had existed before the significant loss. One does not necessarily jeopardize the memory and the tradition of the lost one, but begins to integrate, to assimilate all that was meaningful from that relationship into the developing future.

Death as Birth

Finally, a word about death itself. The family often yearns to be assured that death is not the ultimate end of a precious relationship. "Will I ever see her, be with her again?" There are specific religious answers to this question, but I believe that we humans share an intuition that life does not end with death, that the spirit does not simply evaporate when breathing ceases, that the essentials of one's unique individuality are not obliterated. For some there is the comfort in realizing that one lives on in one's children, one's family, one's work, and the genetic continuity passed on from parents to children.

I would like to share my own strong sense that death is analogous to birth. We tend to attach little significance to birth or the gestation period that precedes it. This is significant because I intend to compare our conscious lifespan to the life of the fetus in the mother's womb. The 9 months of fetal life do not seem impressive in comparison to the normal lifespan. But when one considers that the entire story of evolution on this planet is recapitulated in that brief period, the fetus passing from one evolutionary stage to another in telescoped succession, that 9 months tells a wondrous story indeed. We are not clear whether the fetus possesses at any time before birth a mental state that approaches what we know as consciousness. It is not too outrageous to assume that as birth draws near, some premonition or sensation of a catastrophic event imminent and irreversible might affect that tiny individual, if only as a primitive feeling, different perhaps from previous instances of shifts and changes of position in the mother's body only in the steady, accelerating progression toward the final trauma of which the earlier adjustments had been simply a foretaste.

There are many little deaths in our lifetime. Each opens out to a new threshold, a new beginning, the birth of new worlds one after the other; all are simply a foretaste of the final trauma of death. Is it unreasonably speculative to assume that, again, as before—so many times before—a new world begins at a new level, a new plane? Is it not possible that death as we know it is the trauma of birth into a new, unforeseeable, larger life? One is reminded immediately of the imagery so universal in near-death experiences. Even more dramatically supportive is the abundance of material in religious lore, particularly in Christian scripture and tradition. We must die to live eternally. Baptism, the sacrament of initiation into Christian experience, is regarded as new birth into another order of being fully realized only after death. I remember that, when my own father was dying, he spoke of long-deceased family members all around him; he talked and even sang with them. Hallucination—perhaps. In terms of ''normal'' conscious experience, most certainly. But I see this to be significant testimony, not so strange in the light of a faith that promises reconciliation with those that have gone before. If nothing else, it is a beautiful, curiously appropriate possibility. It is somehow inconceivable that an entity so inherently complex and yet pitifully undeveloped as is the ''mature'' human organism when regarded from a spiritual point of view should simply evaporate to oblivion. It is my belief that family as we know it is comparable to the form of communal life that lies beyond.

References

Adler, A.: *What Life Should Mean to You.* New York, Capricorn Books (1931)

Bice, M.K.: The Healing of the Dying. J Religion Health, July, p. 188 (1978)

Buber, M.: *The Knowledge of Man.* New York, Harper and Row Publishers (1965)

Frankl, V.E.: *Man's Search for Meaning: An Introduction to Logotherapy.* New York, Washington Square Press (1963)

Garland, C.A.: *Psychosocial Care of the Dying Patient.* New York, McGraw-Hill (1978)

Hamilton, M.; Reid, H.: *A Hospice Handbook.* Grand Rapids, Mich, William B. Eerdmans Publishing Company (1980)

Jung, C.G.: *Psychology of Types.* New Jersey, Princeton University Press (Bollingen Series XX) (1971)

Linn, M., S.J.; Linn, D., S.J.: *Healing Life's Hurts: Healing Memories through Five Stages of Forgiveness.* New York, Paulist Press (1978)

Macquarrie, J.: *Principles of Christian Theology.* New York, Charles Scribner's Sons (1966)

Nouwen, H.J.M.: *The Wounded Healer.* New York, Doubleday and Company, Inc. (1972)

Nouwen, H.J.M.: *Out of Solitude.* Indiana, Ave Maria Press (1974)

Rahner, K., Ed.: *Encyclopedia of Theology.* New York, The Seabury Press (1975)

Sanford, A.: *The Healing Light.* Minnesota, Macalester Park Publishing Company (1947)

Schoenberg, I.B.; Carr, A.C.; Peretz, D.; Kutscher, A.H.: *Psychosocial Aspects of Terminal Care.* New York, Columbia University Press (1972)

Tyrrell, B.J.: *Christotherapy.* New York, The Seabury Press (1975)

Westcott, M.R.: *Toward a Contemporary Theology of Intuition.* New York, Holt, Rinehart and Winston (1968)

Whitmont, E.C.: *The Symbolic Quest.* New Jersey, Princeton University Press (1969)

6. The Hospice Care Team

In Chapter 1, we emphasized the need for a comprehensive approach that deals with the patient's medical, social, psychological and spiritual problems over a period of time and in a variety of settings among the objectives of a program for the care of the terminally ill. It is through a multidisciplinary team that hospice care addresses these objectives. In this chapter, we will examine the individual components of the hospice care team and the way in which they are selected, trained and evaluated. Administrative considerations of staff strength, work load and similar matters are covered in Chapter 8.

Advanced malignancy brings with it a variety of problems. In addition, the patient and his family bring to the terminal illness all of the baggage of life, including pre-existing personality, marital and financial problems. In coping with all of these complexities, a team approach is of immense help; it is sometimes necessary to draw upon professional expertise from a variety of fields in order to resolve difficulties. Furthermore, patients are highly individual in their ability to relate to other people; therefore, the availability of many team members provides the opportunity for support from a number of sources. It is not uncommon for the most important emotional support to come from a non-physician member of the team.

It is this feature of hospice that serves as the enabling link between the kind of personal attention which the revered family physician could provide and the sophisticated techniques of modern health care. There are few circumstances left in which it is possible for one kindly and well-trained physician or nurse to provide the breadth and depth of care which a well-organized hospice care team can offer.

Although the strength of a multidisciplinary approach lies in the spectrum of talent it brings to the task, it is most vulnerable in its need for co-ordination among team members. Co-ordination requires both communication and leadership. There must be an opportunity for the various members of the hospice care team to communicate freely regarding each individual patient and about the program in general. Each team member must be able to offer his knowledge and experience and to hear the contributions of others. Various mechanisms can be developed to permit this kind of interchange. The responsibility for co-ordinating the activities of team members rests primarily with the physician. In our own program, the clinical nurse practitioner has been of immense help in assisting the physician with this burden.

An important feature of multidisciplinary care in a hospice program is the lack of sharp distinction between the functions of the various team members. Although each has his area of expertise and primary responsibility, each must be alert to the problems and needs of the patient in other areas. All should share in providing psychological and emotional support to the patient and family. This role is important because team members are in the strongest position to offer this service. It is far better that they do this than that there be a separate "psychological counselor." There is no dearth of people who are willing to volunteer to provide advice to terminally ill patients and their families, but our experience has been that the impact of such counselors is negligible compared to that of the team members who are meeting the patient's physical needs day by day.

Team Members and Their Roles

The details of composition of a hospice care team will vary from program to program. Described below are the roles of the most common team members. The precise makeup of the team in each program will depend upon local circumstances, including program objectives and available personnel. What follows, then, are general guidelines based upon what we have found to be helpful.

For obvious reasons, our emphasis here will be upon those functions that are somewhat different for hospice patients than they are for other patients. Thus, we are looking specifically at the role of each team member in hospice.

Study and reading are very useful beginning points for individual team members to learn about hospice care, particularly if they are to avoid repeating the mistakes of others; however, the bulk of such learning comes from experience. It is only by active involvement in a program that a hospice worker truly begins to see hospice principles and to understand his own particular role.

Physicians

Physician involvement is essential to the success of any program for the care of the terminally ill. In hospice care physician leadership is necessary for the program as a whole and for co-ordination of the team efforts with each individual patient.

Hospice Physician.   We use this term to designate a physician who devotes a significant share of his time to the care of patients in the program. Many hospice physicians will also be immediately concerned with the organization and operation of the program. Physicians may come to hospice work from a wide variety of backgrounds. A hospice physician must be familiar with the principles and practice of hospice care and must have an understanding of oncology. Much of what he needs in these fields, and in pharmacology and other areas which will be important to him in his work, can be learned through experience in hospice work. What he needs to begin with is competence as a physician, the ability to learn, and the personal characteristics which lend themselves to success in hospice work. These are difficult to define, but obviously include compassion, patience, maturity and confidence.

Once involved in the hospice program, the hospice physician will serve as the personal physician for terminally ill patients in the program, directing his attention at palliation and employing the techniques described in Chapter 4. For new patients and for those considering whether or not to enter the program, it will often be the hospice physician who will provide explanations of the hospice concept. The physician member of the hospice team is obviously responsible for the planning and ordering of the patient's medical care. It is he who sees the patient in the context of his prior medical history and who possesses the knowledge of the natural history of the disease process, which is so important to planning medical care. It is he who must make some of the difficult decisions described in Chapters 3 and 4. In order to make hospice care work properly, the hospice physician must be prepared to work with team members from other disciplines, drawing upon their knowledge of other fields and of the patient. He must be prepared to properly deploy and direct the various members for maximum benefit to the patient. He must communicate comfortably with other physicians.

Attending Physicians for Hospice Patients. In the Church Hospital hospice program, a member of the Church Hospital medical staff referring a patient for hospice care has the option of continuing as the patient's attending physician, using the hospice physician as consultant; alternatively, he may simply turn the patient over to the hospice physician. In some other programs, the hospice team serves as a support service in a consultant capacity; the patient, in all instances, remains under the care of the attending physician. In both systems the attending physician is a critical member of the hospice care team. His performance very profoundly affects the success of hospice care. It is important that he be philosophically in tune with the objectives of the program and be familiar with the principles of hospice care. He must be fully and consistently committed to having his patient in the program. He must be able to work with and utilize the hospice care team. It would be nice if every attending physician with patients in a hospice program possessed the personal characteristics and understanding of hospice principles which make a good hospice physician, but it would be unrealistic to expect this. Individualization is necessary, but the hospice care team, including the hospice physician, will sometimes have to provide some of the elements of support and comfort which are not forthcoming from the patient's attending physician. Through constant and continuing education of attending physicians as a group and as individuals, they should increasingly gain knowledge of and sympathy with the principles of hospice care. It is in this way that hospice programs grow.

Referring Physicians. Physicians who turn patients over to the hospice physician and his team are still, in a sense, team members. These physicians need not have a detailed knowledge of techniques in hospice care, but it is imperative that they thoroughly understand hospice philosophy and have a general acceptance of the approach. Although detailed, ongoing reports are not necessary, referring physicians should be informed of major developments with respect to their patients. The avenues of communication should be kept open.

In a hospice care program for the patients of staff members of a single hospital, particularly if it is the first program in the area, the demand for hospice care will be immense. Some physicians who are not members of the hospital's medical staff will refer patients to medical staff members for the sole purpose of making them eligible for the hospice care program. This can create problems if such patients fail to meet the criteria for admission to the program or if the program is overloaded. Medical staff members should be urged either to direct these referrals to the hospice physician or to check with the hospice care staff before accepting such patients.

House Officers. The way in which interns and residents relate to a particular hospice program will depend upon local circumstances, but it is a matter that should be very carefully addressed by program leaders. There are obvious advantages to encouraging house officer participation in hospice programs, but there are some problems that come with this approach.

The advantages are those of disseminating understanding of hospice care to young physicians during their period of specialty training. In addition, the participation of capable, interested house officers enlarges the team's capacities. However, the routine rotation, particularly for short intervals, of interns and residents through a hospice program can result in misunderstandings and misadventures from lack of knowledge about, and sympathy with, hospice care.

It's important that, to the extent that house officers are to be involved, they should be carefully oriented to the elements of hospice care and to their responsibilities. The lack of proper orientation can lead to troublesome frustrations on the part of other members of the hospice team, particularly the nursing staff. Periodic re-education is necessary. For example, the organizational structure of a hospital may be such that the house officer will be the one who is charged with the responsibility for pronouncing patients dead and completing the death certificate. In such instances, he needs to know how to do this expeditiously and unobtrusively. Many families of hospice patients wish to remain with the patient for a while after death; the co-operation of house officers in not dismissing families from the room while the act of "pronouncing" goes on is a small but often important point. Young house officers also frequently have problems with the large doses of narcotics employed for pain control unless they have been provided with adequate instruction. As in other areas of graduate training, physicians should not be expected to provide service without concomitant education.

Nurses

Much of hospice care rests in the hands of nursing personnel. Hospice care draws heavily on the high tradition of nursing; fundamental principles of sound nursing practice are foundations upon which hospice programs are built. The nurse brings to the hospice care team a familiarity with the physical and psychological function of the patient which is critical to making decisions about the patient. Any observations regarding pain, appetite, bowel habits and other symptoms, as well as the assessment of the patient's mood and attitudes, are essential to good palliation. The provision of sound nursing care in the form of positioning, mouth care and skin care are critical ingredients in patient comfort. Nursing personnel in the home care setting may make it possible for the patient to have much of his terminal illness in the familiar surroundings of his own home.

Nursing care in a hospice program is basically no different from good nursing care elsewhere except that it reflects the change in orientation from cure to palliation. However, certain attributes are particularly valuable for the hospice nurse. One must be astute in determining what the patient and his family perceive as needs and problems. One must be able to assess the nature and severity of symptoms, paying close attention to non-verbal signals. Very often patients are reluctant to ask for medication and, as noted in Chapter 4, satisfactory pain control depends upon titration of appropriate analgesic, which in turn depends upon an accurate perception of the patient's pain.

The hospice nurse must possess a sound understanding of hospice philosophy, principles and practice. Often the team member to whom patients and relatives will turn for counsel, the hospice nurse should be comfortable in dealing with problems of impending death. One should be able and willing to leave herself open to questions from the patient and family, responding to them as well as possible and not being unduly discomfited when she is unable to provide specific answers.

The hospice nurse is well advised to be prepared for certain things that occur rather frequently in the care of the terminally ill. Discharge planning often requires a great deal of time. The potential for emotional involvement with patients is enormous. Although hospice care has its satisfactions, the frustrations are substantial and often very graphic.

Since the patient's family is a part of the unit of care in a hospice program, there must be more exacting attention to observation of the family members in order to recognize stresses and conflicts. There must be a greater willingness to intervene for the purpose of providing support and assistance to loved ones than there is with non-hospice patients.

The hospice nurse, in addition to providing direct nursing care, serves a supervisory and consulting role for non-professional workers. One must be alert to lack of understanding or acceptance of hospice principles on the part of other personnel.

As noted below, volunteers are used more extensively and in an expanded role in hospice care. The nurse must accept volunteers and to be able to work with them, and must provide the appropriate balance of supervision and independence for each volunteer.

The special features of home care nursing, as well as some general principles of hospice nursing, are dealt with in detail in Chapter 7. It must be understood that the home care nurses are an integral part of the hospice team. It is only through excellent co-operation between those responsible for nursing care in the hospital and those who handle it at home that true continuity in terminal care can be provided. The home care staff in our program visits hospitalized patients as necessary and maintains constant liaison with the clinical unit nurses and the clinical nurse practitioner.

In our program the clinical nurse practitioner plays a major part in the management of hospice inpatients. CNPs participate in the initial screening of patients being considered for admission to the program and assist in the determination of whether specific patients should be accepted. They are particularly helpful to the hospice physician in this respect because they are familiar with the work load on the nursing unit. They carry out the admission history and physical examination, write routine orders and play a vital part in titrating analgesics for pain control. They begin the patient's nursing care plan. Soon after completing the initial history and physical examination, a CNP sets up meetings with the patient and family to review the goals of the hospice program and to elicit special problems that may exist in each individual case. CNPs see that the patient and his family are introduced to the members of the hospice team with whom they will have contact. Each day a CNP usually sees each patient alone and with family members.

The clinical nurse practitioner maintains communications with the referring physician, the patient's attending physician, other nursing personnel and the various members of the hospice care team. In many respects CNPs serve as the co-ordinator of the patient's care. They monitor his status and make recommendations for adjustments in the treatment program. By virtue of special training and experience, the CNP forms an important link between nursing care and physician care. CNPs usually initiate discharge planning. They provide some of the services performed by house officers in hospitals with residency training programs. In addition to all of this, the CNP is an important contributor to clinical conferences and continuing education programs.

Nursing assistants or aides are a vital part of the hospice team. They are intimately involved in the day by day care of the patient. In developing a hospice program, careful attention should be paid to the proper selection and training of nursing assistants. For the program to function effectively, these individuals must have a knowledge, understanding and acceptance of hospice principles and must possess those personal traits that enable them to work effectively with the dying patient and his family. The unique role which those providing the physical elements of patient care have in meeting the emotional and spiritual needs of the terminally ill has already been emphasized. Patients and families vary immensely in their capacity to relate to various members of the hospice team. Periods of ''opening up'' may be transient and brief, but they are immensely important. The confident reassurance or the gentle touch at the right moment by an understanding aide can sometimes be an irreplaceable therapeutic measure.

Social Workers

The goal of Social Work Service is to help the patient and his family deal with the personal and social problems of illness, disability and impending death. In hospice care this is particularly important. The social worker assesses the problems, needs and capacities of the patient and his family and brings to the hospice team a special knowledge of community resources, which can be of help. All hospitalized hospice patients and their families are seen by the social worker so that the social, emotional, environmental and financial impact of the terminal illness may be evaluated.

A social worker involved in hospice care obviously needs to be familiar with hospice philosophy and principles. He should have a special interest in working with the terminally ill as well as those special talents that make it possible to work co-operatively with a multidisciplinary team. He is involved in the provision of supportive and therapeutic counseling, discharge planning, direct assistance to the patient and his family and in the bereavement counseling. The social worker is one of the team members who is involved with both inpatients and outpatients.

The nature of social work services is in most respects quite similar for hospice and non-hospice patients. Nonetheless, certain differences can be identified. A knowledge of special problems in the dying patient is required for hospice work. There is potential for emotional involvement with patients and their families. There often seem to be less time and less room for error. There is somewhat heavier involvement with other members of hospital staff, particularly physicians and nurses, than there is in dealing with non-hospice patients. In hospice care, the social worker participates more frequently and actively in team conferences and staff development activities. One must be prepared to give more of oneself and to accept less compliance on the part of the patient. Direct patient counseling probably occupies more time than with non-hospice patients and the social worker usually makes a larger commitment of time to the family than is true with non-hospice patients.

Our hospice social worker has found herself doing a number of interesting (and some not very interesting) chores. She often serves as a sort of travel agent for out-of-town family members, arranging for food, lodging and transportation. When family members are fearful of losing their jobs because of time away from work, she speaks directly with employers. She has been to court on behalf of a hospice patient when there had to be a guardianship arrangement and has been involved with juvenile authorities concerning the custody of children after their mother's death.

Dietitians

The approach to nutritional management of the terminally ill patient must be individualized. For example, the patient with a substantial life expectancy may be materially helped by improving his nutritional status, whereas for the patient with a very limited life expectancy this consideration becomes irrelevant.

A profound state of malnutrition and wasting frequently accompanies malignancy and is often the most significant and disabling feature of the patient's disease. Anorexia is often compounded by a perverted sense of taste and smell. Patients frequently say that food just doesn't taste right.

In order to overcome or minimize these problems, the patient's co-operation, to the extent possible, is required. He should be allowed a free choice of types and quantities of food. Special attention must be paid to the appearance, aroma and temperature of food. Portions should be small, with frequent snacks. Families can often provide special ethnic foods that may stimulate a lagging appetite. The patient should never be forced to eat. Although augmentation of basic diet with supplemental feedings may in some circumstances be helpful, it must be remembered that a diet is only beneficial to the patient when the prescribed diet is individualized to meet the needs of the particular patient.

For some patients, considerable dietary manipulation may be advisable in order to improve nutritional status relatively early in the course of their terminal illness. Diet supplements may be useful. However, later in the course of illness emphasis should shift away from maintenance or improvement of nutritional status and should be directed entirely at patient comfort. The dietitian must therefore maintain communication with the physician and nurses so that she is familiar with therapeutic objectives of dietary management at any given time.

The social aspects of food should be kept in mind. Appetite is often poor when patients are eating alone, so arrangements should be made for guest tray service if at all possible. Light food and liquid refreshments should be available on a complimentary basis for the patient's family. Birthdays, anniversaries and special events can serve as an occasion for a celebration, with patient, family and staff sharing together.

Thus, although special diets for therapeutic purposes are seldom necessary, the dietitian must be constantly alert to the often changing dietary preferences of the patient and be ready to suggest alternatives when foods become unappealing. An individualized dietary care plan should be based on the dietitian's assessment of the appetite, food preferences, tolerances and the physical capabilities (chewing, swallowing, ability to feed self) of the individual patient. This requires periodic discussion with the patient and his family; there is no substitute for observing the patient at meal time. Conferences with other members of the hospice staff regarding the patient's nutritional care and possible need for changes in diet can be invaluable.

Pharmacists

In hospice care, drugs are used both in conventional and unconventional fashions and dosages, particularly in pain relief; it is important that the hospital pharmacy staff be conversant with principles of hospice care. Certain agents such as high-dose morphine solution, Dilaudid suppositories and artificial saliva are seldom used in non-hospice patients.

For work with outpatients, it is often helpful for a hospice program to involve at least one private pharmacy outside the hospital. The pharmacist there should be thoroughly oriented to hospice care and be considered part of the hospice operation. It may be advisable, incidentally, that the identity of such a pharmacy be kept secret or at least not be publicized, because of the problems that arise when a pharmacy is known to stock substantial amounts of narcotics. The selected pharmacy should provide emergency and delivery services. The pharmacist needs to be imaginative in the preparation and packaging of materials for hospice patients.

Physical Therapists

The physical therapist can be of significant help to a number of hospice patients. His value should not be overlooked in establishing a hospice team.

The aim of physical therapy in hospice care is in actuality somewhat different from its aim in other patients. For non-hospice patients, the objective of treatment is usually improved function, but usually for hospice patients the objective is relief of discomfort.

Again, individualization is necessary; it depends upon the particular patient and the stage of his disease. The goals of the physical therapist are usually to help the terminally ill patient adapt to his physical limitations and to permit him to function at his highest possible physical level. An effort is made to maintain function as long as possible. While doing this, it is important for the physical therapist to provide emotional and psychological support, for as the patient's condition deteriorates he often becomes increasingly concerned about his lessening ability to perform the activities of daily living. Generally speaking, the physical therapist will find it helpful to allow the hospice patient to talk more than other patients and perhaps to use recreational therapy more frequently. In addition to his role in working directly with the patient, the physical therapist must be prepared to offer his professional assessment of the patient's functional status and physical capabilities.

Because of the somewhat different orientation of physical therapy for hospice patients, not all physical therapists are suited to this type of work. It is generally best that one member of the Physical Therapy Department be selected for this role. The prime requirements are a special interest in working with the terminally ill, the ability to work co-operatively with the multidisciplinary team, adaptability, and some knowledge of the issues of death, dying and grief. Naturally, the physical therapist must have an understanding of and agreement with hospice care principles.

The physical therapist must be prepared for a level of emotional involvement with hospice patients which is seldom achieved with non-hospice patients. He must be willing to accept the fact that the overall course of hospice patients is one of deterioration, rather than of rehabilitation and improvement. He must be ready to discontinue physical therapy when, in his judgment, it is clearly no longer helpful or in the patient's best interests.

Within this framework, the techniques employed are much the same as they are for non-hospice patients. Certain measures such as chest physical therapy and breathing exercise can be particularly helpful.

Psychiatrists and Psychiatric Nurses

Hospice programs have varied in the extent and manner in which they have utilized psychiatric services. In our program, staff psychiatrists and the psychiatric liaison nurse are available to hospice patients, as they are to other patients in the hospital. They have been used in the evaluation and management of problems of a truly psychiatric nature occurring in terminally ill patients and their families. In this role they have been most helpful. However, we do not regard dying itself as a psychiatric disorder. As pointed out in Chapter 4, we have generally felt that, except in unusual circumstances, straightforward psychological support to patients and family members in handling serious illness and impending death is best provided by members of the hospice care team who are immediately involved in meeting the physical needs of the patient.

Other hospice programs have, of course, used psychiatric support services much more liberally in planning, policy making, patient care and staff support. Psychiatrists have played a critical role in the development and implementation of some hospice programs. Several psychiatrists at the International Hospice Conference sponsored by St. Christopher's in June 1980 argued persuasively for the inclusion of psychiatrists in all hospice care teams. They felt that by virtue of their training and experience psychiatrists provide special skills of value to terminally ill patients, their families and the staff caring for them. It was their opinion that the psychiatrist should be a member of the hospice care team, rather than a detached consultant as described above. They noted that each hospice group should design its own approach and choose the most appropriate staff and also recognized that psychiatrists with the requisite skills were not available to all hospice groups. However, they recommended that every effort be made to recruit suitable psychiatrists into all programs.

Obviously, each developing hospice program will have to make its own decisions with respect to the role of psychiatrists. That decision will be based largely upon local circumstances.

Chaplains

By the nature of their function in the hospital, chaplains often play a critical role in hospital-based hospice care. Chaplains have been deeply engaged in most hospice programs. Their ministry is available to all involved in hospice care. In addition to providing spiritual support to the patient and family in an unusually demanding situation, the chaplain must be alert to their physical and psychological needs.

Primary attention is to the spiritual needs of patients and family. ''Spiritual'' is used in its broadest sense and must be distinguished from specific religious concerns. The distinction is important in order to respect the wishes of those persons who do not profess or care to align themselves with a religious affiliation. Those who do wish to receive religious ministrations such as the sacraments are accommodated appropriately.

The chaplains routinely visit hospice inpatients and see hospice outpatients as appropriate, often through referral from the home care staff. Contact is established with the patient's own clergyman where indicated. As can be readily appreciated, other members of the hospice staff often play a role in the spiritual aspects of hospice care, so that the chaplains make themselves available as a resource to the staff. In this capacity they help the staff to deal with difficult questions which patients and families may raise. They also help the staff to deal with pressures and stress and, as a consequence, enable them to expand and deepen their own capacity to provide excellent hospice care.

When the chaplain functions as sole pastor for the patient and family, he may be asked to officiate at the funeral upon the death of the patient and to participate in bereavement follow-up. Patients and their families should be encouraged to attend and be made welcome at regularly scheduled services in the hospital chapel.

Because of their interest in and knowledge of the hospice program, our chaplains have played a variety of other roles. They have participated in staff training and continuing education and are available for educational activities in the community. They also assist the Director of Volunteers in interviewing and evaluating recruits for positions as hospice volunteers.

For hospitals that do not have a chaplain, the appointment of a volunteer or part-time salaried chaplain co-ordinator from the community should be considered for the hospice program. There are several possibilities for locating such a key person.

Most communities have a ministerium, which is usually ecumenical and fairly representative of the clergy in the area. Some are more effective or representative than others. Appeal can be made to such a ministerium for help in identifying a suitable candidate for hospice chaplain co-ordinator. It can also be helpful to identify the clergymen in the community most distinguished for strong pastoral ministry; these may not be the most popular or celebrated clergy. This person or persons could be invited to participate, along with key representatives from the hospice program or committee, in locating a suitable chaplain co-ordinator.

Prerequisites for a position as chaplain co-ordinator include strong commitment to the program, highly developed pastoral skills (marked by a caring and loving nature), flexibility so far as ecumenical considerations are concerned (this would require a good understanding of traditions other than his own), leadership ability (which would include the respect of other clergy in the area), strong counseling experience and some background in health care (particularly with regard to the needs of the dying and their families). Such a candidate must be a person with whom the staff is comfortable and in whom staff members have confidence. Interviews with the medical director, administrative co-ordinator, social worker and at least one member of the nursing team should be required.

The chaplain co-ordinator would recruit suitable clergy from the community to assist in hospice chaplaincy on a regular, shared, scheduled basis. These clergymen would be on call during particular times during the week and be responsible during that time for regular visits to the hospice patients and families. These chaplains should be considered members of the hospice staff and should be utilized as such for consultation, referral, education and voluntary attendance at staff meetings.

The chaplain co-ordinator or chaplain is expected to participate regularly in staff sessions and preferably should be included in the hospice committee or governing agency for the hospice program. He is held accountable for the chaplaincy service; like other members of the team, his performance is regularly observed and reviewed.

Volunteers

In most hospice programs, volunteers have played a vital role. Not only does the volunteer offer a perspective that is difficult for the professional to achieve, but the presence of volunteers makes it possible to offer some services that could not otherwise be provided. They have in actuality made some hospice programs financially feasible. Volunteers are of immense value both to the hospice inpatient and in the home care setting.

The difference in function between hospice and non-hospice care is generally much greater for volunteers than it is for other members of the hospice team. For the other team members, most of the change is one of degree and emphasis. For the volunteer, there is usually a fundamental change, in that direct patient care and contact is introduced. As a consequence of this there is an enormous increase in responsibility. The nature of hospice care not only permits this shift but encourages and capitalizes upon it. In a few hospitals volunteers are already being given a larger role in the direct care of general medical-surgical patients. This practice has, however, not yet become widespread outside of hospice programs.

Hospice volunteers can be effectively used to provide physical comfort measures for patients. Naturally, the question arises as to the degree to which volunteers may be permitted to provide such services. A good rule of thumb is that the volunteers can safely and productively take on all of those chores that would be assigned to the lay caregiver in the home. This includes the clean-up and bathing of the patient, back rubs, changing beds, getting the patient up in a chair, Foley catheter care and certain aspects of charting, such as intake and output records. Utilizing the volunteer for such duties for the inpatient not only makes it possible for the nursing staff to extend services to patients which would otherwise not be available, but it also permits the introduction of some flexibility in ward routine. For example, it may be difficult for nursing personnel to provide a bath for a patient who wishes one at 2:30 in the afternoon, but this can often be done by a volunteer.

In utilizing volunteers for the provision of physical comfort measures, it is important to take into account the individual preferences of volunteers and to supply adequate training and supervision. Volunteers vary immensely in their interest in performing direct physical care; no volunteer who finds such work unappealing should be forced to provide it. In this connection, incidentally, there is an appreciable difference between the need for such service on day and evening shifts and it is sometimes worthwhile to take this into account when making volunteer assignments. Careful, thorough training in each technique and appropriate supervision are as important for the volunteer as they are for the professional or the family member.

In addition to physical comfort measures, the volunteer can provide a number of psychological services that are of critical importance to the hospice patient. As has been noted elsewhere, these seem to be accomplished more effectively by those who are otherwise directly involved in the patient's care than by individuals especially assigned for these purposes. Such measures include listening, explaining the nature of the program, serving as a conduit to the proper professional members of the hospice team, taking walks around the hospital to places like the chapel, being available at the time of death and participating in the provision of bereavement support.

By virtue of their status as non-professionals, volunteers are sometimes in a better position to offer certain direct patient services than are other members of the hospice care team. They serve as bridge between the world which the patient knows outside the hospital and that which he finds within its walls. Without interrupting the discipline and routine of the nursing unit, volunteers can sometimes soften its edges.

The volunteer is often seen by the patient and his family as someone outside the normal health care delivery system and they are thus sometimes willing to share thoughts and feelings which they do not wish to express to other members of the team. The volunteer's freedom from other hospital responsibilities often permits him to listen and talk with the patient at a critical juncture when the patient is transiently willing and able to open up and be receptive.

A key word in the proper use of volunteers is *balance*. There is a need for a proper balance between volunteers and professionals as they work side by side. Volunteers may need to earn the respect of their co-workers by demonstrating their interest and responsibility. Professionals must be ready to help and be willing to provide respect when it is earned. There must be a clear understanding of what is expected of volunteers. Effective teamwork comes from having a common goal and a commitment to achieving that goal. Finally, there is a need for balance in the amount of supervision which is given to volunteers. Too much supervision is stifling and discouraging to the volunteer, but inadequate supervision is unsafe. The extra effort made by professionals to enable volunteers to contribute pays rich dividends not only to the hospice team, but most importantly to the patient and his family.

It is apparent that recruitment of volunteers is vitally important to the program. In an era of generally declining volunteerism, most hospice programs have found that volunteers are available. The work is interesting and rewarding, but even more appealing to many volunteers is the willingness of hospice programs to give them responsibility. Talks by staff to groups interested in working with the dying can be added to the traditional methods of recruitment, such as newspaper articles, church bulletins and referral by staff employees and active volunteers. In our own program we have a number of nurse volunteers and one retired physician volunteer.

The next section of this chapter deals with the selection, training and evaluation of hospice personnel in general, but most attention is directed to the professional team members. Because of the importance of, and difference in, selection and training of volunteers, a few observations are in order here.

Screening of volunteers is crucial to the program. Each applicant should be interviewed by the Director of Volunteers and at least one or two other members of the hospice staff. Our chaplain serves in this function. For a volunteer with a professional background, there is a further interview by a hospice staff member from that particular discipline.

Criteria for selection of volunteers should be established. In our program we have only three rigid criteria. A high school diploma is the minimum educational requirement. Prospective volunteers are asked to commit themselves to the program for at least one year. It is our policy not to accept anyone who has experienced the death of a close family member within the past year. We purposely use only a few criteria in order that we might achieve maximum heterogeneity among our volunteers. We feel that diversity is an important attribute of the volunteer group.

Unquestionably, intangibles and subjective considerations play a role in the evaluation of prospective volunteers. Nonetheless, there are certain characteristics which experienced workers responsible for selecting volunteers find to be reliable predictions of performance in care of the terminally ill. Basically, we are looking for well-integrated individuals who want to give and care. A calm and comforting disposition and ability to communicate are valuable attributes. The volunteer should be able to serve patients and families from different cultural and religious orientations. Older individuals who are retired from a busy work life are a fertile source of volunteer strength. Preoccupation with death and manifestly unresolved or immature attitudes toward death are extremely undesirable characteristics in a volunteer. The very subjective individual who tends to become overly involved or the individual who tends to impose his own values upon others can be a liability, as can the insecure, erratic and impatient.

Eliciting evidence of the existence of these various traits is simple in some instances and may require the most skillful use of interviewing techniques in others. The judgments of the interviewers may be imperfect. For that reason, volunteers, like all other members of the hospice team, should be appointed on a trial basis and their performance should be carefully monitored during their probationary period.

Experience has shown that properly selected volunteer workers can be quickly trained to perform a variety of simple direct patient care functions safely and effectively. The training program for hospice volunteers should be very carefully prepared and should be conducted primarily by hospice team members. Lectures, class discussions and outside reading should all be used. Once a certain amount of basic material has been covered, on-the-job training under the supervision of professionals and volunteer members of the hospice team should be initiated on the nursing unit and in the home care setting.

Our 20-hour classroom program for volunteers is coordinated by the Nursing Staff Development Office. It includes the following:

1. Attitudes toward death and dying—chaplain.
2. Grief and bereavement—chaplain.
3. Disease processes and effects of therapy—hospice physician.
4. The hospice concept—hospice physician.
5. Symptom control—clinical nurse practitioner.
6. Inpatient hospice care—head nurse.
7. Outpatient hospice care—home care director.
8. Nursing procedures—staff development nurse.
9. Social services in hospice care—social worker.
10. Role of the volunteer in hospice—senior volunteer.

Once the volunteer has completed formal training and a probationary period, the director of volunteers and other senior members of the hospice staff should keep in touch with the volunteer and obtain feedback on satisfaction and performance. A regular meeting of the hospice volunteers to provide educational opportunities and emotional support is valuable and the volunteers should attend regular staff meetings at which patients, policies and other matters are discussed. The volunteer thus serves as a full-fledged team member.

Other Needs, Other Answers

Terminally ill patients and their families not infrequently present problems that require the specialized techniques and knowledge of professionals from areas other than those described above. One of the advantages of a hospital-based program is the relatively ready availability of such individuals, even though they may not be, in the strictest sense, members of the hospice care team. The enterostomal therapist, for example, can often be of immense assistance, not only to the patient with a poorly functioning colostomy, but also in the treatment of decubitus ulcers and intestinal fistulae. For some head and neck cancer patients, the speech therapist can offer useful assistance. We have been pleased by our early experience with art therapy. The music therapist can also be helpful. There are other members of the hospital staff, such as housekeeping and maintenance personnel, whose contact with hospice patients is, for the most part, casual. For all such individuals a brief basic orientation to hospice philosophy and practice can be most worthwhile.

In our program we have not, up to this point, utilized physicians' assistants in hospice care. However, they obviously can be valuable members of a hospice care team (Kuhrts, 1977). Their function is similar to that of clinical nurse practitioners, working both with inpatients and outpatients.

To be truly comprehensive in its care of the terminally ill, the hospice care team must be prepared to draw upon all available resources to meet the needs of patients and their families.

Staff Selection, Education and Evaluation

KATHLEEN ROCHE, R.N., M.A.

Selection

No matter what other attributes a hospice program possesses, it is, in the last analysis, only as good as its staff. It is surprising therefore that very little has been written about the criteria for and process of staff selection.

Four qualities seem to be of utmost importance for staff members; these are competence, sensitivity, flexibility and maturity.

Competence. Professional competence is of tremendous importance. This is particularly true for home care staff, who work with minimal supervision and opportunity for immediate collaboration in their day-to-day patient contact. For all hospice workers, assessment skills must be highly developed. Naturally, as an individual gains experience, capacity for accurate diagnosis and effective intervention will increase. Nonetheless, there is no substitute for a high level of professional competence even as a staff member begins his work as part of the hospice care team.

Sensitivity. Hospice care was born out of a holistic need for low technology and high caring. Sensitivity is the very foundation and fabric out of which hospices are made. The person who chooses to work in hospice must have done so out of a personal desire to serve, to experience and to grow. While it is recognized that the staff member will to some extent meet some of his own needs as he attempts to fulfill those of others, those responsible for selecting hospice staff must be on the alert for manifest or hidden agendas, such as proselytization, resolution of previous guilt or grief or acquisition of personal gain.

Sensitivity is a key requirement which affects all levels of the program. If a hospice team is to be durably constructed its members must integrate hospice principles into their own attitudes, caring not only for their patients, but also for each other and for themselves. The concept cannot survive unless the team is alert and its members are available to each other in times of need.

Sensitivity is somewhat intangible and abstract; it is difficult to define. Yet it conveys a sense of activity rather than stagnation. One is reminded of the story of the "warm fuzzies" in which the recipient learns he can replenish his supply only by giving it away. As a hospice staff member learns to trust his intuition and to act upon it, he gains confidence in himself and in his ability to meet those very subtle needs that can so greatly enhance the quality of living and dying. This positive feedback encourages the development of even greater sensitivity. In other words, not only must staff members be selected in part because they possess sensitivity, but also that sensitivity must be nurtured throughout their hospice experience.

This process requires mutual trust, understanding and patience. Advanced development of skills and attributes are acquired over time, but their potential for development can be readily detected by a sensitive administrator. In a hospital-based hospice, the hospital administration must not only approve of the hospice philosophy, but also must actively encourage the development of new skills and techniques that enhance humanistic care in general. Sensitivity training, popular in the '60s, may be a valuable tool to assist the staff in coping with the intimacy experienced in hospice care.

No one will deny that sensitivity and caring together with a high level of competence are vital to humanistic health care. Each potential staff member must be evaluated for these talents, but alone they are not really enough.

Flexibility.   Hospice care requires the courage to deviate from the safe and conventional. It demands a willingness to improvise and an ability to adapt.

In a sense, fear of change is related to fear of death, the ultimate change. If a staff member maintains his or her security by following the letter of the law, by ritual or by a repetitive care plan, he may feel extremely anxious in a setting that strives to individualize patient care. A secure, imaginative individual, on the other hand, will feel fulfilled in an environment that not only permits, but also encourages, flexibility and creativity. The point is that an effective hospice staff member should not only be capable of being adaptable but also should enjoy it.

Maturity.   Maturity may be difficult to define, but it can usually be sensed; it is an important attribute for the hospice team member. It is related to age and experience, but it is not limited to these components. One's philosophy of life, death and after-life is important in maintaining balance through difficult situations, such as the death of a favorite patient or many patients in a short time. It is also critical to the maintenance of a sense of priority during times of stress or fatigue. Staff members should be able to admit mistakes in order to learn from them without fear of hard reprisal. They should accept responsibility for their actions and behavior. They should be capable of owning to their own feelings and be willing to practice forgiveness of themselves as well as others. Those who cannot do these things have no place in a high-caring milieu. They will contaminate it.

In addition to the above four attributes, there are a number of other features of staff selection which should be commented upon. In selecting hospice staff it is important to look for individuals with varied personal and professional experience. In other words, one should aim for a team with some heterogeneity. This process not only insures expert care for a larger variety of patients, but also expands the perceptions and attitudes of the staff. For example, a nurse with strong psychiatric experience can have her dormant medical-surgical skills refreshed by a nurse who is strong in these areas, while teaching and sharing her psychosocial skills. The whole staff will become more holistically oriented.

The ability of staff members to function dependently as well as independently is important. Some hospice functions require the capacity for acting on one's own, whereas others demand integration in team activities.

Some attention should be given to the history of the hospice applicant's life experience. Frequently, an individual who has experienced a loss in his own life and has coped well is not only sensitive but also less anxious (Kübler-Ross, 1975). In a sense he has been there and has survived; he is an excellent role model for the family. On the other hand, a newly-bereaved individual who has not had the time necessary to develop his coping and distancing would seem to be at high risk for serious stress problems.

No one is entirely exempt from occasional disturbing guilt feelings when his patients die. This is especially true when several patients die in a short period of time, suddenly or unexpectedly. A staff member with a low self-image may be plagued with serious doubts in such circumstances, much to his own as well as the program's detriment.

Because there has been some misunderstanding about it, one attribute which does *not* seem to be of any importance in selecting hospice staff nurses deserves mention. This is the type of educational background. There is no place for educational prejudice or for blanket rules regarding possession of a specific type of degree in the initial appointment of staff nurses. The important focus must be on what an individual can bring to his patients. Theoretical background which may be lacking can easily be made up by a motivated individual.

It is probably wise to make all appointments to the hospice staff on a trial or probationary basis. Transfer into other types of work environment should be easy and graceful if things do not work out for an appointee.

Similarly, seasoned hospice personnel may at times wish a temporary transfer for a change of pace, as well as environment, and to permit some re-education in other areas. It is worth pointing out that this may be extremely difficult to accomplish for the home care staff, since experienced temporary replacements are almost impossible to find. For home care staff, some type of contractual arrangement outside of the home care department may allow for the provision of back-up service during such temporary reassignments or during vacation and sick leave. An occasional change of duties may prevent an immense amount of wear and tear. Thus a staff member may assist with teaching new personnel, students and visitors or may take on some administrative functions. For qualified workers who enjoy public speaking, there are usually numerous lecture requests that can be assigned. Imaginative innovation in deployment of staff is very helpful in keeping the staff fresh, happy, relaxed and effective.

Education

Orientation. Orientation of new staff needs to be as flexible and individual as the care plans of the hospice patients. It should consider whether the employee is new to the organization, to hospice care or to particular aspects of hospice care. The orientation will aim to supplement the individual's knowledge and clinical experience. Most staff members will require fairly basic education and training in the fundamentals of hospice care. Although this must include some theoretical background, much of the training must be practical and experiential. It is only when intellectual knowledge meets emotions and feelings and becomes integrated and congruent that the hospice education is complete; this is a never-ending process. There really is no substitute for an experienced mentor working one-to-one with a new hospice staff member. This not only results in highly individualized instruction with immediate feedback, but also provides some anxiety-reducing support.

Orientation should include education on matters relating to death and dying, palliative care, hospice concepts, pharmacology, concepts of pain control, local policy, nursing procedures and other matters particular to the area which the staff member is entering. For example, an experienced general medical-surgical nurse entering the home care program will be provided with instruction and techniques of home visitation, as well as an introduction to thanatology, grief and bereavement and stress reduction. Pedestrian topics such as automobile first aid and self-defense may prove very useful for a home care nurse. Staff input into the orientation process of new employees is extremely valuable.

Because there is a practical limit to the amount of individualization that can be provided in the initial orientation, it will be necessary in most hospice programs to set up a basic instructional course that includes some classroom instruction, which can then be supplemented by individual instruction on the nursing unit or in the home care situation.

Continuing Education. Hospice care is not a "once-trained always-trained" proposition. There is need for continuing education. This can be accomplished in a number of ways. Regular conferences utilizing cases available in the program are an extremely valuable teaching tool. This often needs to be supplemented by periodic topic-oriented instruction covering such matters as the control of specific symptoms, techniques of dealing with grief reactions and new methods in tumor control. There is great value in sending staff members off from time to time to other hospice programs and to hospice meetings. Maintaining an up-to-date indexed list of recommended readings can be very helpful.

Within the structure of a hospice program, someone responsible for planning, organizing and executing initial orientation programs and continuing education programs can be very helpful. Such an individual must, however, draw upon all members of the hospice team for input into the educational process.

Evaluation

No hospice program meets its full potential unless there is careful evaluation of what is being done. This should be done for individual hospice patients and for individual hospice staff. The precise method of evaluation is a local and individual matter depending upon the particular program. The method chosen should strike a balance between the formal and systematic, on the one hand, in order to insure completeness and fairness; it should be individualized, subjective and supportive, on the other hand, in order to insure the maximum benefit from the evaluation process. Evaluation for hospice staff can be a time for honest feedback, as well as a creative sharing and setting of goals and expectations for the immediate future. Each staff member brings his unique gifts into the hospice experience. The evaluation process presents the opportunity to acknowledge these attributes and to clearly inform the staff member how these relate to the hospice program in general. Naturally, praise breeds a positive atmosphere for continued good work; it needs to be administered in regular doses rather than saved for a yearly overdose.

The evaluation process can often be a useful two-way street. Staff members need to be actively involved in program development and policy making. Their practical day-to-day experience and awareness of trouble spots can be extremely helpful in obtaining the maximum from the program. Furthermore, when staff is involved in the development of guidelines and policy, they are more likely to understand their rationale and to comply effectively. Evaluation should be careful and honest but to the extent possible it should be carried out in a non-threatening fashion.

Staff Stress—"Burn Out"

Stress is a normal part of life. Life without stress is devoid of an important dimension. Stress can be a positive factor leading to growth and progress. It can also be paralyzing and can contribute to illness (Selye, 1956, 1974; Pelletier, 1977).

Throughout the medical care system there are many sources of stress and many stressful situations. The care of the terminally ill in general, and hospice care in particular, can be the source of both beneficial and harmful stress for personnel.

We will be looking here at the harmful aspects of stress among members of the hospice care team. In hospice care, as in some other areas, this goes by the term "burn out." Although some feel that problems of staff stress and burn-out in hospice care have received more attention than they deserve, it would be unrealistic to overlook it as a potential source of difficulty for the hospice care team.

It is important to recognize that everyone is prone to the harmful effects of stress; many people are reluctant to admit this propensity or to recognize the unfavorable effects of stress when they occur. Conversely, for some the *fear* of stress can in and of itself be anxiety-producing and enervating (Shealy, 1976). Once staff stress occurs, it tends to be contagious. This is not the place for a detailed consideration of the cause, prevention, recognition and treatment of psychological stress syndromes, but it is worthwhile to make certain observations with respect to staff stress among the hospice care team.

Causative Factors

There are a number of factors in hospice care which foster the development of unfavorable stress reactions. The day-in, day-out close contact with dying patients brings the hospice worker into frequent confrontation with his own mortality. In such a setting it is difficult to avoid contemplation of one's own death. A hospice team member's unresolved concerns in this regard provide a fertile ground for stress reactions. Furthermore, for individuals with a background in the health professions, death does indeed convey an element of defeat which, even in the absence of unresolved fears, can be a source of frustration.

Many hospice care workers tend to be idealistic. Some adopt an unrealistic view of what it is possible to accomplish for the terminally ill. The discrepancy between their expectations and reality can be the source of severe disappointment and distress.

The nature of hospice care deprives team members of some very effective and comfortable defense mechanisms in dealing with terminal illness and death. Depersonalization, detachment, clear definition of responsibility and stereotyped response can be most helpful when one is threatened by the death of a patient. However, hospice care is characterized by a high degree of personal attention and involvement, lack of strict role definitions for team members and an emphasis upon flexible and innovative responses to situations (Pelletier, 1977). These, and a number of other factors, added to the usual stress-provoking aspects of medical care, make the hospice team member particularly prone to staff stress.

Effects of Stress

Excessive stress leads to a number of undesirable effects. For the individual team member, unpleasant symptoms of anxiety, sleeplessness, and loss of appetite can be most troublesome (Flynn, 1980). The net result of these symptoms is depleted energy and concentration. These in turn lead to impairment of the team member's capacity to provide excellent patient care. In addition, intra-staff friction may develop between team members, which again is both unpleasant for the individuals involved and harmful for patient care. Finally, unhealthy stress responses lead to a high turnover rate among hospice personnel; this not only results in considerable dislocation for individual team members, but also impacts unfavorably on the quality of care provided to patients.

Prevention of Stress Reactions

Prevention of staff stress is more satisfactory than is its treatment. Prophylaxis is not always possible, however, and every mature hospice care program has experienced some adverse stress reactions. It is important, however, to take certain steps to minimize their incidence.

The selection process for team members is important and deserves the careful attention of program leaders. Mismatching a person and his job can create an environment favoring the occurrence of severe stressful reactions. It is best to avoid appointing to hospice teams individuals with clearly unhealthy attitudes toward death and dying. People vary immensely in their capacity for physical work and psychological stress; work assignments should take these variables into account.

Once staff members have been selected, proper orientation can be a valuable tool in preventing staff stress. Each team member should understand hospice principles and practices. He should accept the hospice approach and should comprehend the way in which he fits into the team. Most important, however, he should be given a realistic picture of what it is reasonable to expect to accomplish in the care of the patient terminally ill from malignancy.

Hospice program leaders should create an environment in which team members are able to help each other deal with stress. Mutual sharing and assistance among the members of the hospice care team are probably the most effective weapons in the prevention of harmful staff stress reactions. There must be ongoing efforts at communication between team members. Regular meetings of the hospice team play an important part in this respect. Top-flight educational programs encourage personal growth, which in turn enhances personal satisfaction. Patient care conferences not only provide an improved sense of understanding about individual patients, but, if properly conducted, also permit the venting of some concerns, fears and feelings by team members.

Certain team members are particularly suited to the provision of support to other team members. The chaplain and the psychiatric staff come immediately to mind, as does the hospice physician. However, the important point is that *all* team members feel responsibility for the welfare of their teammates and feel free to draw from other staff members for help as they need it. The creation of this kind of environment takes time, but it is well to begin with this as a goal.

The experience of hospice programs with group conferences designed specifically for staff support has been variable. Many programs have found such meetings extremely helpful. Others have not been favorably impressed with their value; they have made the staff support function a byproduct of conferences whose primary objective is education or patient care. Regular inservice education programs which update staff members' knowledge can help reassure them that they have done all they could as caregivers.

If meetings for the specific purpose of staff support are held, they should be organized with extreme care. The leadership should be thoughtfully selected and the programs carefully monitored to be certain that their effect is positive rather than negative. Poorly planned or poorly conducted meetings of this type can be most detrimental to the effective function of the team.

It is usually advisable to assign hospice workers to regular shifts over a period of time. Periodic short breaks from work should be provided and vacations should be given and taken. When a hospice staff member is away from work, his time off should be completely free of hospice responsibilities and concerns. Staff members should be encouraged in the development of outside interests. They should be instructed in the use of some distancing techniques that are compatible with hospice care philosophy. It is important that they learn to use their colleagues effectively in the care of patients. Each hospice staff member must recognize that he is indeed a member of the team, that he does not individually need to provide all aspects of care to each patient and that he can call upon his teammates for help. It goes without saying that the physical structure of the environment is important in avoiding stress, fatigue and frustration.

Individual staff members can themselves take some measures that may prevent or reduce stress. Various self-regulation techniques have been recommended. Some effective conventional modes of coping with stress are regular exercise or other diversionary activity, good eating habits and adequate sleep. While such measures obviously promote health and well-being, they are particularly important for caregivers who may habitually think of the needs of others and rarely of their own.

Stress management can also include such innovative techniques as yoga or eliciting the relaxation response through biofeedback (Brown 1974, 1977). Progressive relaxation of bodily parts, rhythmical breathing exercises or meditation by means of focus of attention and concentration may allow the stress response to decrease and are said to be effective coping tools when taught and used properly (LeShan, 1974; Benson, 1975; Carrington, 1977).

If the logistics can be worked out, it is often helpful to develop a system whereby hospice staff members can arrange temporary transfer to other types of work. This not only assists in avoiding staff stress, but also encourages cross-fertilization between the hospice program and other providers of patient care. Some programs have found it advantageous to have a regular rotation system. If this is not possible, temporary or permanent transfer should be made easy and graceful.

With respect to staff stress, it is important to note that the integration of hospice patients into a general medical-surgical nursing unit, as has been done at Church Hospital, alleviates some of the stress problems related specifically to terminal care. Under this system each team member has responsibility both for hospice patients and for patients who will recover. In this environment, staff stress problems more nearly approximate those of general medical-surgical care. Nurses, for example, may be frustrated by the end-of-shift feeling that, because of time constraints, they were not able to accomplish as much in the care of some of their patients as they would have wished. Some have been reluctant to recognize the role in which other members of the hospice care team can play for the patient whose need simply is just to have someone with him.

Although the sources of stress in this type of program tend to be more those of a general nature than those which are related specifically to terminal illness care and death, the hospice team members are still thrown into intimate contact with the dying and their families. They are, therefore, subject to the individual sense of loss in specific cases which is a feature of all hospice care. Nonetheless, it has been our impression that the overall effect of the integration of hospice patients with general medical-surgical patients has been to diminish staff stress problems.

Recognition and Treatment of Staff Stress Syndrome

Both for the individual team member and for the hospice team as a whole, it is difficult to draw a clear-cut line between a healthy stress response and a frankly abnormal or pathological state. *Extreme* stress in the individual and the team can be easily recognized by the disintegration of function. However, next to prevention of harmful stress reaction, early recognition and prompt treatment are the optimal means of preventing serious difficulty. Each hospice program should develop its own mechanisms for the rapid and appropriate diagnosis and treatment of stress. The nurse, for example, should understand her responsibility to detect signs of staff stress in personnel and to report these to nursing management.

In the individual team member, symptoms of harmful stress reaction include fatigue, sleep disturbance, anorexia, somatic symptoms without organic basis (e.g., headache and diarrhea) and withdrawal (Patrick, 1979). Depression, anxiety and anger may occur. The use of depersonalizing and derogatory terms for patients is frequently seen. Errors in observation and recording, together with decreased concern about mistakes, may be a symptom of unfavorable stress reaction.

Treatment of staff stress syndrome in a team member must be highly individualized. In some instances, simply a little informal counseling by another appropriate individual such as the head nurse or chaplain may be the wisest choice. More formal counseling may be necessary for others. Sometimes staff stress symptoms in the individual will respond to relatively minor modifications in assignment, routine or schedule. Occasionally, temporary or permanent transfer out of the program provides the only solution. The decision as to whether or not to employ psychiatric therapy for team members suffering from work-related stress must obviously be made on an individual basis.

Staff stress tends to be a communicable disease. A relatively minor degree of stress among individual team members may mushroom as the team interacts. Therefore, one must be alert to team symptoms as well as individual symptoms. No staff functions entirely smoothly at all times, but a sharp change in the level of intra-staff friction and frequency of personality clashes deserves the attention of program leaders. So does an unusual number of requests for transfer. Some observers have commented upon the fact that an increased pace of activity with an appearance of frantic bustle may be a sign of group staff stress.

Once the early symptoms of an unfavorable staff stress syndrome are recognized in the hospice team at large, treatment consists fundamentally of amplification of the preventive measures. Potential causes of unhealthy stress reactions should be sought out and dealt with appropriately. Sometimes such sources are physical factors in the environment, workload distribution or institutional regulations. Sometimes an individual team member is a source of team stress; stress is indeed contagious.

Beyond eliminating, insofar as possible, the causes of team stress, everything should be done to facilitate the capacity of staff members to help each other. The regular staff meeting schedule should be examined to determine whether the frequency and the quality of the meeting is adequate. Some consideration may be given to the development of special programs for staff support, although, as noted above, these must be developed carefully, not casually. Scheduling the provision of breaks and vacations and the easy opportunity for temporary or permanent transfer must all be looked at.

There is no simple, uniformly effective treatment for staff stress either in the individual or in the team. The important points are as follows. It can be more easily prevented than treated. The potential for occurrence of staff stress should be recognized and the program designed and operated so as to minimize the opportunity for it to develop in the individual or in the team as a whole. However, because prevention is not infallible, the mechanisms for early detection and treatment should be established.

References

Benson, H.: *Relaxation Response*. New York, Avon Books (1975)

Brown, B.: *New Mind, New Body Biofeedback, New Directions for the Mind*. New York, Harper and Row (1974)

Brown, B.: *Stress and the Art of Biofeedback*. New York, Bantam Books (1977)

Carrington, P.: *Freedom in Meditation*. New York, Doubleday Anchor Books (1977)

Flynn, P.: *Holistic Health: The Art and Science of Care*. Bowie, Md., Robert J. Brady Company, Prentice Hall Publications (1980)

Kübler-Ross, E.: *Death as the Final Stage of Growth*. New York, Prentice Hall Publications (1975)

Kuhrts, S.B.: Symptom Control in Terminal Disease. P.A. Journal Vol. 7, 189 (1977)

LeShan, L.: *How to Meditate*. New York, Bantam (1974)

Patrick, P.: Burnout, Job Hazard for Health Workers. *Hospital*, p. 87–90, 1979

Pelletier, K.: *Mind as Healer, Mind as Slayer*. New York, Dell (1977)

Selye, H.: *The Stress of Life*. New York, McGraw-Hill (1956)

Selye, H.: *Stress Without Distress*. New York, McGraw-Hill (1976)

Shealy, N.: *Ninety Days to Self Health*. New York, Bantam (1976)

7. Outpatient Hospice Care

KATHLEEN ROCHE, R.N., M.A.

If a man's home is his castle during life, it should remain so as he faces death. Traditionally, man was born and died at home—often the same one. He was cared for by people he knew, loved and trusted in this familiar environment. He maintained control over his domain.

The modern trend in health care has been hospitalization of patients so that the high technological advances of the last decade can be applied to the fullest extent. High technology, however, cannot replace the human caring that is so vitally needed as earthly life draws to an end. Home care most frequently meets the needs of the dying person who has family to care for him. Additionally, it provides opportunity for the family to anticipate the loss of a member and to interact in an intimate and satisfying way. The proverbial house can be put in order, business finished and peace made as necessary (Jivoff, 1979). This period of shared grief tends to enhance the bereavement period.

While the benefits of home care make it superior to other available options for both patient and family, it is a difficult commitment to make; it requires deliberation, thought and careful planning. Home care is not a panacea effective for everyone. The choice must be made by the entire care-providing group; most especially, the patient must participate in the decision.

The hospital-based home care program is perhaps the ideal system of hospice care because of its flexibility and continuity. Both emotional and physical support can be provided whether the patient is in the hospital or at home. Even in the home setting the health care team has the resources of the hospital on which to rely if necessary.

In general, home care serves the patient's medical, social, economic and spiritual interests by extending health care to his residence. In addition to providing continuity of care, the home health program shortens the length of hospital stay and in some instances obviates the need for hospitalization. This in turn promotes appropriate utilization of beds and other hospital facilities and reduces health care costs. Home care provides the opportunity to continue or to modify patient teaching begun in the hospital. Factors in the home environment which may interfere with top quality patient care can be identified early and corrected. The

125

home care program serves as an excellent setting in which students and health care professionals can be taught holistic family care and hospice philosophy; they can test their clinical skills under a supervisor (*Church Hospital Home Health Policy Manual*, 1981).

The whole population benefits from humanistic health care practices. Because the patient and family are an interacting system, holistic practice dictates that they be treated as a single unit. Each member affects the other, as does any change in family status. Thus an adolescent son may experience crisis when his father's terminal illness forces him to sacrifice or delay college education to assist in the provision of care or to supplement the family earnings. The entire family's strengths, weaknesses, resources and responsibilities must be taken into consideration as care plans are devised. Too often only one individual's wishes are taken into consideration. Usually this is the family leader or most verbal member. The best hospice care will be sabotaged by a frightened or angry family member who has not been taken into consideration in the plans.

Reimbursement for hospice services is at present relatively uncertain and the subject of some debate. For home care in general, there are an abundance of regulations with which providers must comply if they are to be reimbursed; at this time there are relatively few regulations specifically for hospice care. In Maryland, for example, most of the specific regulations were established in connection with the Blue Cross hospice demonstration projects which began in September 1979. These regulations are largely the same as those for any of the coverage packages which contain home care benefits for the insured. However, benefits are extended to include coverage of medications and one continuity visit to smooth the transition between home care and institutionalization. One bereavement visit to the family following the patient's death is also covered by the pilot program. The purpose of the coverage for one visit is to permit evaluation of the family needs and the making of referrals to the appropriate community resources. A major problem to date has been the sparsity of community programs for the bereaved or widowed.

Hospice home care for Medicare and Medical Assistance patients must comply with the usual regulations for these programs. Thus only skilled intermittent services (nursing and other) to *homebound* persons will be reimbursed. Hopefully, the homebound stipulation will, at some future time, be waived for hospice patients. If symptoms are truly controlled and the philosophy of helping patients and families to live to the fullest is upheld, occasional outings and socialization are possible for many hospice patients and should not disqualify them from reimbursement. Furthermore, if patients can conserve their limited energy by having their conditions monitored in the comfort and convenience of their home, rather than engaging in lengthy and strenuous travel to physicians and hospitals, they may be able to take part in outside socialization, family outings and short trips. The breaks in the sickness routine serve to elevate the morale of all concerned and leave behind some pleasant memories for the survivors.

Pre-authorization of equipment (such as hospital beds and wheel chairs) and visits by the Medical Assistance Program may take weeks; this is longer than life expectancy for some hospice patients. The problems are complex ones involving ethical issues such as the allocation of relatively scarce resources. The answers to these questions are difficult, but dying patients are a minority group whose rights and needs deserve attention.

The Church Hospital Home Care Program

Our Home Care Program was originally developed as a public health nursing experience for the students in the hospital school of nursing. Although the school closed several years before the hospice program officially opened, home care remained viable and was under the direction of Helen Fowler, R.N., until her death. By this time, Home Care had progressed to the status of a full-fledged department within the hospital structure. The preliminaries of certification were well under way when a new full-time Home Health Director was hired. In January 1979, the program was certified for Medicare and Medicaid and additional nursing staff was hired. At the present time the staff is composed of five registered nurses, two home health aides and one secretary. All positions are full-time. There is also one three-quarter-time volunteer secretary. The program handles non-hospice as well as hospice patients.

Four of the R.N.'s do patient visiting; the fifth serves as director. Naturally, if clinical emergency situations arise, the director does do patient visiting. Administrative visits are also made for supervisory purposes.

At the start of the program only professional staff was used. Now that the program is more highly developed, home health aides have been utilized. Personnel will be added as needed as the program grows.

To date we have not been able to accept into the program certain patients whose physical needs have been greater than could be met with our staff or volunteers. These include people who have insufficient caregivers to provide round-the-clock care or who require more than five visits a week on a prolonged basis.

Until quite recently, a medical social worker served the home care patients by contractual agreement. The cost of indirect services, however, became prohibitive; they represent about twice the time involved for the actual visit and are non-reimbursable by third party payors. A method of having one hospital social worker serve hospice patients both at home or while hospitalized is being developed. It is hoped that such a plan will not only reduce cost, but also provide greater continuity as well.

Our experience with physical therapy was just the opposite. The Physical

Therapy Department itself was a young, developing department. Serving the home care patients proved too great a burden on the department. A contractual agreement has worked out much more effectively. Speech therapy is required for less than 5% of the home care population and it has been most satisfactorily provided through contract.

Because the program is hospital-based, each of the hospital departments can serve the home care patients. Thus, pastoral counseling, nutrition therapy, respiratory therapy, etc. are all available when needed. Therefore, the home health department does not have to duplicate personnel already employed by the hospital to serve patients at home.

Durable medical goods and pharmacy service are also provided by contract. The pharmacist is an integral member of the team. Not only does he monitor the drug profiles carefully and stock the specialty items, but he also frequently makes up special suppositories for use when patients can no longer swallow. This service often makes it possible to keep patients at home; their families are not traumatized by having to administer injections. The pharmacy delivery service is much more than a convenience. It saves human energy and relieves the nursing staff of the temptation of assisting families by bringing the drugs themselves. For safety reasons, it is wise for the staff not to acquire the reputation of transporting drugs (especially narcotics) or otherwise controlled substances. The nurse should not risk personal harm unnecessarily.

A letter of agreement with a large local ambulance company insures continuity of care should hospitalization become necessary. City and county ambulances will transport patients only to the nearest hospital. It is imperative that the patient return to Church Hospital rather than to another where he and hospice care are both unknown. Thus traumatic, aggressive or invasive treatment and drug withdrawal is avoided. Ambulance drivers are alerted if a hospice patient is to be transported so that they will not initiate resuscitation.

The *primary nursing concept* is utilized by the home care department. Each nurse carries a caseload of patients and plans their nursing care in collaboration with the attending physician. Since one nurse is responsible for each patient, long- and short-term goals can be well planned and accountability issues are more clear. The department is open only Monday through Friday, 7:30 A.M. to 4:00 P.M.; there is a nurse on call every day. This means that each nurse not only has the responsibility for a caseload (usually 12 to 17 patients), but also must become familiar with the total population. To accomplish this, there is a weekly meeting on Thursday morning during which time each nurse gives a complete report on each new admission and an update on the rest. Occasionally, the primary nurse will form a special relationship with a patient and family and choose to be notified by the on-call nurse if a special patient's death is imminent. Because all nurses experience such a relationship, they understand the request and do not feel their competence is threatened. Rarely does a primary nurse or patient request a change of assignment, even during long or repetitive admissions to home care. Changes of assignment usually require sensitive handling for all parties concerned to avoid or deal with feelings of inadequacy or abandonment. Program experience has taught us that the hospice patient's visit often consumes 50 to 100% more time than that of other patients. In general, there are more bases to cover in a shorter period of time because of the shorter life expectancy. Patients and families simply cannot and should not be unduly rushed during this period of crisis. Admission visits for *all* patients generally require double the usual visit time, since the patient care plan data base must be obtained on the initial visit.

The Church Hospital program extends its general home care boundaries to serve a greater area for hospice patients. It is important, however, not to require of the staff more than 20 to 30 minutes driving time. Clustering visits saves staff time and reduces cost of travel.

One of the strongest features of the Church Hospital program is the guarantee of a bed for an emergency hospice admission. Families are less fearful of attempting home care if they have the back-up support of an inpatient bed. The home care nurse's anxiety is reduced by the awareness that there are standing orders to be followed should management problems which cannot be successfully dealt with at home be observed.

Advantages and Disadvantages of Hospice Home Care

Home care is nothing new on the health care scene. In this era of high technology and impersonal health care, it has been rediscovered and newly appreciated. The following advantages of home care should be noted:

- The cost is considerably less than that of institutional care and is reimbursable either in part or totally by some health insurance plans.
- The family and patient have the opportunity to fully experience the final days as a family together without any restrictions except those they wish to impose.
- The patient and family retain much more control over the situation; feelings of hopelessness and helplessness are greatly reduced.
- Invasive life-prolonging (or death-prolonging) procedures are unavailable in the setting but can be obtained if needed. They are less likely to be inappropriately used in a crisis.
- Food and activity can be geared toward usual life style or preference.
- Hospice staff can help teach a family how to care for the ill person, monitor progress and be available for problems or questions.

- Hospice staff, entering into the family system, has the opportunity to effect positive change in the patterns of communication and guide the family toward resolution of conflict.

Disadvantages to be considered are these:
- Families often do not understand how demanding the 24-hour care of a person can be; they can become exhausted.
- Reimbursement of cost is often to some extent uncertain.
- Families may feel abandoned by the health care system and improperly prepared for the task of home care. Emergencies can trigger overwhelming anxiety.
- Unless the care is planned, the bulk of nursing responsibilities may fall upon the shoulders of one person, who becomes drained (Roche, 1980).

The critical consideration is, however, that the care settings may not be so important as the caring that takes place within them. Home care should not be forced on anyone. Very apprehensive people may respond to the opportunity to meet with the primary nurse several times before they are actually placed under her care. On-call systems, readmission policy and use of emergency staff visits should all be explained several times to allay anxiety.

Family meetings can be used to elicit feelings, as well as for teaching and planning purposes. Children often benefit greatly from having the opportunity to voice their concerns and ask questions in the group setting. Some families, especially if they are large, may benefit from opening and closing the meeting together as an entire unit, while breaking into adult and child subgroups, each with an experienced hospice team member, for part of the meeting. As with any group, it is most difficult for one facilitator to pick up on all the important issues and it is impossible to properly supervise a split group. At least two experienced members of the hospice team should be present for a family group meeting. Facilitators should be comfortable with the normal emotional expression that often accompanies the discussion of such a painful situation as the loss of a family member. While specific stages are not necessarily individually identifiable, anyone facilitating a family conference should be familiar with Dr. Kübler-Ross' five descriptive stages of dying. (Kübler-Ross, 1969).

Hospice Screening and Acceptance Procedure

In the Church Hospital hospice program, all patient referrals are first directed to the Home Health Department. Since the anticipation is that many patients will be cared for at home after a brief period of stabilization of symptoms as inpatients, home care planning is a logical starting point. The referring physician is asked to submit sufficient information to permit an evaluation of the patient. In the Home Health Department, a determination is made as to whether the patient meets the admission criteria. In addition, insurance policies are evaluated, nurses' caseloads balanced and questions answered. Following this general screening, medical screening is conducted by the nurse practitioner. The final decision regarding acceptance of the patient is made by the hospice physician, Dr. Bernard Yukna, who also serves as the Home Care Medical Director.

After an outpatient has been accepted into the program, the hospital admitting office is contacted and given the information necessary to reserve a bed and make the appropriate identification plate if hospitalization is required. Direct admission to the inpatient unit can then be accomplished. Long or uncomfortable delays in processing information are avoided.

Similarly, for a patient who is already in the program and on home care for whom readmission is required, the primary care nurse can provide the admitting office with the necessary information; admission can thus be accomplished expeditiously.

Preparation to Return Home

Preparation for discharge from inpatient hospice care is really begun during the screening process before admission to the program. Rapport has already been established with the Home Health Director or her designee. Rounds are made at least every other day to check patient progress in anticipation of discharge to home care. Home health staff, together with the physician, nurse practitioner, social worker, discharge planner, patient and family meet to discuss any equipment which might be needed.

Patient care teaching is done in the hospital by the staff and volunteers. Refinements are made in the actual home setting. Since there is constant communication between the home care department and the nursing unit, the initial visit at home can be scheduled the same day as discharge if necessary. Some patients realize that they are going to die very soon and want to be at home. These are times when discharge must be successfully completed very quickly to fulfill the patient's request. It is essential that the contracting agencies with which the hospice deals understand the priority nature of assisting the patient to get home. The family has to be well prepared and understand that the patient in such a situation may only live a few hours. If they are unprepared, they may fear that they caused the death prematurely because of their inexperience. The importance of alerting the on call-nurse to the discharge of such an ill patient cannot be overemphasized. She needs not only the usual appropriate clinical information, but also directions to the house by the quickest route as well.

Families are encouraged to keep a simple notebook "chart" on the patient. This is especially important if many caregivers are going to be involved with the patient. Sometimes it is appropriate to photocopy the patient care plan from the home health record for the family. Care must be taken to document the updates in the official record as well as on the family chart. Through this notebook, the nurse can be kept abreast of changes noted by all family members, not just the one present during the visit, or to pick up on information which a single caregiver may forget to report. One can also write out the instructions. On-call staff also finds this helpful. The most important point is to keep the notebook chart *simple*. If it is packed with medical and nursing jargon, the patient and family may be intimidated by it and not use it.

Many patients want to maintain as much independence and control as possible. Others become forgetful, confuse medications and need help. In either case, a supply of small bottles into which the day's doses have been individually poured and marked with the appropriate administration time is most helpful. Many patients set an alarm clock to remind them of their next dose. Preprocessed medication doses are a must during the night. They allow the patient to have the proper dose of medication without having to fully awaken and disrupt sleep.

The importance of bowel care cannot be overemphasized. It seems that many patients have to experience the discomfort of severe constipation and/or impaction to fully understand the need for prevention. All too often patients protest that they do not need stool softeners or laxatives that are ordered because they have never been constipated in their life. Analgesics, particularly narcotics, given in large quantity over a prolonged period quickly change usual bowel patterns. The care plan is not complete or effective until the patient and family are thoroughly indoctrinated about this. Of course, the patient maintains the right to refuse any medication or treatment.

Families often ask what they need to care for a patient at home. Most patients need very little in the way of major equipment. Many do need to rent a hospital bed so that they can be turned, positioned and cared for properly once they are bedbound. Some patients remain ambulatory to the end. The following equipment is listed together with its use as a guide for families. It represents an *optimum*. Where resources are limited patients can, for example, be adequately cared for with two sets of sheets. Very anxious families often tend to overprepare and gather too many supplies (Roche, 1980).

Equipment List

This equipment list is given simply as a guide. Every caregiver quickly develops his own style and favorite patient care products.

Equipment	Use or Underlying Reason
1. Rented hospital bed	To allow for safe lifting and turning without back injury. If total care, consider an electric bed; only the charge for a regular hospital bed will be reimbursed in most cases.
2. Bed care utensil set, consisting of plastic cup, denture cup (if dentures used), kidney (emesis) basin, bath basin, bed pan, soap dish, water pitcher and tray	These items allow caregiver to have all items necessary for personal care readily available. Patients may take these disposable-type sets home from the hospital, since they have paid for them.
3. Five or six fitted bottom sheets	The smoothness of the bottom sheet protects the skin from extra friction and wrinkles.
4. Two large pillows, two medium pillows and one or two small ones with two changes of pillow cases	Pillows are used not only under the head, but also to support the patient's back in a side-lying position. Pillows should also be placed where bony prominences rub, like knees or ankles.
5. Ten flat top sheets	These sheets can be folded in half and used across the middle third of the bed to serve as a turn sheet in moving the person, as well as to prevent bottom sheet from having to be changed should the bed become wet or soiled.
6. One bath blanket or large heavy towel	Use this to keep person warm during baths or procedures.
7. Six bath towels; six wash cloths	To dry patient when bathing; to wash patient when bathing.
8. Six hand towels	For use to put across patient's chest and keep it warm while bath blanket is pulled down to hips to expose abdomen. Also used in feeding patient as a large napkin/bib.
9. Large piece of plastic	Use across middle third of bed and tucked under mattress *under* the turn or draw sheet.
10. Good lubricant lotion for massage; powder	For use in skin care to prevent skin breakdown.
11. Tooth brush, tooth paste, mouth wash	For mouth care.
12. Small table (like card table)	Place care items which are used daily on it for handy access.
13. Rented wheelchair	To allow patient to sit up and be able to get around house (if level), or outdoors.
14. Comfortable chair and other chairs for visitors	To allow patient to be out of bed and also enjoy visitors.
15. One box flexible straws	These bendable straws permit easier drinking, since they adapt to the angle of the patient's head position in relation to the glass.
16. One bag disposable bed pads (Chux). Incontinent patients will use considerably more	Protects bed from soiling.
17. Large size disposable diapers (several boxes) for incontinent patient	To absorb urine; reduces skin irritation and protects bed.
18. All customary personal care items: brush, comb, deodorant, razor or other shaving equipment, cosmetics	The patient needs all his usual favorite products within easy reach.

Equipment	Use or Underlying Reason
19. Television, radio or other favorite diversion	Diversion helps people to relax and pass the time more easily.
20. Spiral or loose leaf notebook with dividers	Handy for recording medications, progress notes, observations and questions for the doctor; categorize each section for locating information easily and rapidly.
21. Trash can with plastic liners and sealing wires	For sanitary disposal of waste.
22. Rented over-bed table or lap tray	For meal tray.
23. Large tray on which complete meals can be served	Allows one trip to be made to bedside and all food to arrive at appropriate temperature.
24. Easy access to laundry facilities	This will permit frequent washing of linen, washed in a way that is most gentle on patient's skin (use of mild detergents, avoidance of starches, double rinses if necessary and use of fabric softeners).
25. Stubby thermometer, one bottle ethyl alcohol, cotton balls, lubricant	From time to time it may be necessary to take the patient's temperature. This thermometer can be used for oral, rectal or axillary recording provided it is thoroughly cleaned after each use.
26. Rented alternate air pressure mattress and pump for bed patients, or egg crate mattress	This prevents or relieves constant pressure on skin, which could cause bedsores.

(Roche, K.A., 1980. Adapted from actual clinical experience in home care, and American Red Cross Home Nursing Text, 1963).

The Process of Home Care

It is the primary home care nurses' responsibility to plan and deliver high quality care for hospice families in the home. This includes writing care plans, keeping accurate records and assisting patients in attaining all the benefits to which they are entitled. These nurses co-ordinate care with consultants and teach and counsel the family caregivers. They must have the maturity and experience to work independently as well as interdependently, as necessary. The role is not easy, but it is most fulfilling.

On admission to home care, baseline data about the patient and his family are obtained and assessments are made as to strengths and weaknesses. This is often done with the assistance of the social worker. Nursing assessments are carried out and problems identified. Teaching home care management of symptoms is continued from the hospital setting. The family is oriented to home care and instructed in how to contact the nurse, etc. Most importantly, the nurse and family relationship is established. There is usually a short period of testing before trust is gained. The nurse wonders if she can trust the family to call with questions before they get into a troublesome situation; the family may call the nurse with minor problems to test the effectiveness of the on-call system. This period is usually short, as all parties concerned are eager to work with each other as they see the positive rewards of symptom relief. The initial visit is often twice as time-consuming as the maintenance visits. Much teaching about patient care is done on a regular basis on each visit as care plans are adjusted. Every effort is made to keep communication as open as can be tolerated and to elicit active patient/family involvement in care planning.

This relationship grows and extends to include the entire family and hospice care team. Families are taught the basics of home care of the patient and are prepared for changes in condition. Preparation is important so that unexpected events do not develop into crises and in order to keep staff and family stress as low as possible. Equipment and medications must be readily available. There is no sense in extending service to the home if the staff is left impotent in an emergency situation. Written instructions (a care plan) to follow are just as important for the family as "orders" are for the nurse. There is always the alternative of admitting the patient to the hospital if this is the most appropriate measure.

Preparedness is based on clear communication. Time spent together during the death trajectory is of little value unless it is used well. This period of terminal care can be a time of growth, shared preparation and marriage completion. Used badly, it can be a time of mutual destruction and can mar memories of relationships. Fear and grief, even if intellectually denied, remain physically active. Despite the presence of these strong emotions, traditional psychiatric therapy is of little value. People respond better to caring and understanding (Parkes, 1978).

Researchers Weisman and Worden (1975) studied the positive effect that mutually responsive relationships had on length of survival. Clearly, the interaction between staff and patients is likely to play a major role in survival. Home care itself may motivate a patient (Sutton, 1979). Similarly, Gielen and Roche (1979) observed that patients who were surrounded by supportive families had not thought much about suicide. Conversely, patients abandoned by support systems not only had suicidal thoughts, but also planned what situations they would act upon.

Clear communication is blocked by such obstacles as double messages and incongruency of body language and speech. Language can be thought of as a way of creating a representation of one's world together with one's perceptions, the choices one sees, hears and feels are available and the means by which one conveys it to others. Thus language is a kind of territorial map of a person's reality. A personal filter system can enrich or impoverish perception and therefore one's reality territory. Unclear images of the world block perception and therefore the choices available (Brandler and Grinder, 1975). Those working with hospice families must be sensitive and alert to these reality maps. Imperative to the helping process is listening to words like "never," "always," "should," "ought," "can't" and "impossible." These, together with patterns of thought that generalize, distort or delete information, tend to narrow the possibilities. Such clues to perception present the opportunity for gentle challenge to expand perception. For example, a cancer patient who makes the statement, ''I want to die because it is impossible to live like this,'' can learn a whole new form of reality by his involvement with the choices of hospice.

The role of the counselor is that of a sounding board, listening and understanding yet ready to reverberate with encouragement, comfort and praise (Parkes, 1978).

Outside support systems such as the national organization Make Today Count (MTC)[1] are most helpful in complementing the hospice support. Most families wish to retain affiliation with their usual support groups. Unfortunately, as the word of the patient's prognosis is spread, old friends and acquaintances often do not feel they know what to say or do; consequently, they distance themselves from the patient. A self-help group such as MTC composed of patients and families with whom there is a commonly shared bond can be an uplifting source of help. Hospice volunteers are of immense importance in weaving a fabric of instant specialized support.

The Home Death

Few experiences in life are more significant than death. Many families, believing that the event will be awful and traumatic, do not consider seriously the option of the patient dying at home. Through the whole process of the hospice concept of care, many families choose to have the patient die at home. Fear and anxiety are reduced as people realize death is more a gradual process than an unanticipated sudden event.

Families are encouraged to communicate with the patient as to his wishes about burial arrangements. Funeral directors have been most helpful and understanding when they were consulted in advance of the patient's death. They have policies and procedures regarding home death from which they are prepared to deviate with hospice families. They must be assured that the patient has been under the care of a physician who can sign the death certificate. Funeral directors tend to remove the body of the deceased from the home quickly in home deaths because so often families, in a complete state of shock in sudden death, do not feel comfortable otherwise. By contrast, however, the hospice families tend not to view the death as an emergency to be dealt with immediately and want to call

---

[1] For more information on MTC and the nearest chapter contact MTC, 1109 Franklin Street, Burlington, Iowa 52601. (There are over 250 chapters in the USA.)

extended members back to the house for one last goodbye. They often wish to bathe or groom the body, sit in silence or pray together and there is no reason the request should be denied.

Even with preparation by hospice care, the event cannot be fully anticipated in advance. In fact the family may expect to avoid grief or mourning through having cared for the patient. No matter how adequate the coping, few people expect the death *now,* at this moment. It always comes as a surprise. An advantage of preburial planning is the avoidance of having to function at a high level while in a state of shock (Director, 1979).

Often the hospice nurse is present at the time of death or shortly thereafter, having been called by the family. Her role is to guide the family through previously made choices, but not to assume functioning for them. The ritual of burial and its planning and preparation are necessary to begin the healing process. Often the first task is to assist the family in the disposal of the patient's medications and equipment. The process of their disposal is symbolic of the recognition that the suffering process has ended. Clothing and mementos can be handled at a later date. If a special relationship has developed among staff and family, closure might be effectively accomplished by the staff member's attendance at the funeral.

Bereavement Visits

The purposes of bereavement visits are:
- To assess the coping ability of the survivors.
- To encourage and facilitate the expression of feelings regarding the loss.
- To reassure survivors that this process, although painful, is normal.
- To identify disturbed, delayed or pathological patterns of grief and make appropriate referrals for long-term followup.
- To give opportunity for the bereaved to examine the process of their increased growth and maturity through the death experience.
- To provide opportunity for feedback about program effectiveness (*Church Hospital Home Health Policy Manual,* 1981).

The visit should be low in profile and aim to reassure (Parkes, 1978). Someone familiar to the family is usually the visitor of choice, since rapport is already established. However, the use of a new visitor, so that the family has opportunity to tell the story again, has been proposed (Lattanzi, 1979). Proper timing of the visit is probably more valuable than delaying or omitting a visit to wait for a particular person to accomplish it.

St. Christopher's Hospice has identified seven categories of bereaved persons who are at special risk following the patient's death. These are:

- Persons of low socioeconomic status.
- Housewives without employment outside the home.
- Those with young children at home (who may themselves be at risk).
- Those without a support system, or those with a family who actively discourages expression of grief.
- Those who show a strong tendency to cling to the patient before death and/or to pine for him afterwards.
- Those who express strong feelings of anger or bitterness before or after the patient's death.
- Those who express strong feelings of self reproach (Parkes, 1978).

Since many of our patients are retired, elderly and on fixed incomes, a different set of criteria are used as guidelines to identify at-risk bereaved:

- Those with a short period of time from diagnosis to death or a violent death.
- Those who have experienced multiple losses in a short period of time.
- Those without a previously established support system.
- Those survivors in poor mental or physical health themselves (*Church Hospital Home Health Policy Manual,* 1981).

Ideally, every bereaved family should have a visit. This is the most appropriate way to evaluate the patterns of coping after the death has occurred, since data gathered prior to the mourning process may be invalid. There is also wisdom in asking a patient who is open to discussion what problems he might expect, from whom, and how the hospice team might be helpful. Patients take comfort in the knowledge that their families will continue to have hospice contact after their death, as well as in sharing such information, which may be of extreme importance.

Dependence on the team should not be fostered, however. This is just as inappropriate as abrupt withdrawal. A type of behavior modification plan in which continued support becomes conditional upon the bereaved person moving toward a new set of goals may be most appropriate. The usual model of the more needy the person, the more attention given needs to be reversed (Parkes, 1978). This process can be effectively and gently accomplished by a statement such as, "Call me when you make your plans," (get a job, etc.).

Bereavement notes should be kept in as detailed a fashion as clinical notes. Periodic audits will indicate patterns which may be useful in treating future families. Information such as length of stay on program, attending and referring physicians, primary nurse, place of death, quality of bereavement and number of visits indicates which physicians tend to refer too early or too late in the disease process. Place of death and readmissions to hospice may indicate which nurses are more comfortable with home death as well as those who are sensitive to the family's inability to cope. Inservice programs and individual guidance can then be designed around these issues.

Discharge from Hospice

A brief note is in order regarding the types of discharge from hospice. The most frequent and obvious is, of course, by death. There are others, however, such as by referral. This category would include situations in which the patient goes to live with an out-of-state relative or wishes to resume aggressive treatment. Similarly, refusal of service or non-compliance with treatment occurs. While these are relatively rare, they do happen. There is a final gray area in which the patient goes into remission. In the Church Hospital hospice program, patients in remission are kept on the program and visited only monthly. Phone contact is made in between visits.

References

American National Red Cross Home Nursing Text. (1963) 7th ed. New York, Doubleday (1963)

Brandler, R.; Grinder, J.: The Structure of Magic. Palo Alto, Calif., Science and Behavior Books (1975)

Church Hospital Home Health Policy Manual: Philosophy and Objectives. Unpublished document (revised January 1981)

Director: Preparing Today for the Eventual Tomorrow. pages 12–21 (1979)

Gielen, A.; Roche, K.A.: Death Anxiety and Psychometric Studies in Huntington's Disease. Omega, Vol. 10, 2 (1979–1980)

Jivoff, L.: Home Care and The Quality of Life. Ed. by E. Prichard, New York, Columbia Press (1979)

Kübler-Ross, E.: On Death and Dying. New York, Macmillan (1969)

Lattanzi, M.: Bereavement Case Manual. Boulder, Colo., Boulder County Hospice, Inc. (1979)

Parkes, C.M.: Psychological Aspects. In The Management of Terminal Disease. Ed. by Cicely Saunders. Chicago, Ill., Edward Publication, New York Medical Publishers, Inc. (1978)

Roche, K.A.: Sharing the Experience of Death: A Manual of Family Care. In press

Sutton, K.: Hospice. In: Make Today Count. Montgomery County, Maryland, Chapter Newsletter, p. 4 (January 1979)

Weisman, A.D.; Worden, J.: Psychosocial Analysis of Cancer Death. Omega, Vol. 6, 61 (1975)

8. Administration of a Hospice Program

GLORIA R. CAMERON, M.H.A.

This chapter addresses the organizational structure, financial aspects and staffing of a hospice care program. It is written from the perspective of a hospital-based program and draws on the experience of the Church Hospital hospice. While the advantages of a hospital-based program are emphasized, the success of other program models should not be ignored. The applicability and appropriateness of any particular delivery mode is contingent upon numerous factors which must be appraised in each community. Many of these factors are explored in the text that follows.

Organization

Questions of how to organize and deliver hospice care in the United States frequently prompt controversy concerning its proper place in the *existing* health care delivery system. The organizational structure needed to support a hospice care program must provide for a very special integration of program components into this system. Whether this calls for an entirely new element within the system or adaptation of existing elements, or both, has not been determined. Continuity of care, which is essential to the hospice concept, is a major medical goal in this country. The organizational challenge posed by this goal can be met by the successful implementation of hospice care.

Church Hospital chose to offer hospice service as a program of care integrated into its existing organizational structure. This approach began with analysis of the components of hospice care as they would relate to the hospital's mission, goals and mode of operation. The approval and support of the Board of Directors of the hospital were procured early in this process.

A review of basic components of hospice care included recognition of the terminally ill patient and his family as the focus of care, the palliation of disease symptoms, supportive efforts in a holistic approach to health care and an emphasis on home care. These characteristics do not preclude the provision of hospice care by hospitals. While they are not necessarily typical of hospital care, there is no reason why they cannot be and many reasons why they should be. In fact, the ability of hospitals to co-ordinate health care resources enhances the potential for delivery of hospice care in this country. As a centralizing entity, the hospital is in a key position to foster continuity of care with efficient use of resources. It was from this perspective that Church Hospital developed its hospice care program.

The structure needed to manage and implement the program and co-ordinate the interdisciplinary team already exists in the community hospital. Hospital accreditation standards require the establishment of an organized medical staff with bylaws and a means of accountability to the hospital's governing body. A standing committee structure typically provides the mechanism for review and evaluation of medical staff practice and functions. These committees are also responsible for providing direct medical staff input and guidance to important medical functions within the hospital (e.g., Pharmacy and Therapeutics, Blood Utilization Review, Infection Control).

This familiar hospital structure is an excellent vehicle to centralize the various hospice care components through formation of a standing Hospice Care Committee. Such a committee derives its authority from the medical staff bylaws and is accountable to the medical leadership and, ultimately, the governing body of the hospital. Representation by responsible hospital management (i.e., administration and appropriate department heads or supervisors) taps the authority of the existing managerial hierarchy and utilizes effective channels of communication. The composition of such a committee will necessarily vary as dictated by the particular organization of services and functions in a given hospital. Representatives would likely include department heads from social work, volunteer activities, home care, chaplaincy, selected nursing supervisors and the administrator responsible for program coordination. Physician members would typically include an oncologist, a family practitioner and any others with special interest or experience in hospice care. At Church Hospital the medical director of the program chairs the committee with other physician members including representatives from the Medical, Surgical and Gynecological services and the medical director of Home Care. Responsibilities of the committee include initiation and review of policies, procedures and forms, evaluation of program status and planning.

Operational choices for hospital-based programs range from establishment of a distinct unit, to an integrated unit to dispersement of patients throughout the facility with services provided by a consultative team. Hospice home care services may be provided by a hospital-based department or through formal liaison with an outside home health agency.

The alternative of a separate unit with designated staff normally presents a prohibitive expense to the typical community hospital. This model is more appropriate in a larger facility or university teaching hospital where institutional organization and patient volumes may support the expense. Another option, that of providing a consultant interdisciplinary team with patients dispersed throughout the hospital, may not effect the desired change in patient management. While the concept is excellent, hospitals may find such a program difficult to co-ordinate; there may be insufficient impact upon the traditional curative environment. This alternative has been successfully employed in some hospitals; the roving consultative team can be an excellent means by which to introduce hospice care to the medical community and may be used as a first step toward the development of a more centralized program.

In the case of the hospice care program at Church Hospital, patients are admitted or transferred to a particular nursing unit in which the personnel specialize in the care of the terminally ill. Other medical/surgical patients are also located in this 50-bed nursing unit. Hospice team members relate to the unit and to the Home Care Department, which is closely aligned with the program. The hospital opted to develop its own home care agency in order to facilitate continuity of care and insure strong control and co-ordination of the hospice program. The Home Care Department also serves non-hospice patients and meets other community needs.

Development of liaisons with independent home health agencies has been accomplished by other hospital-based programs, but presents a difficult management problem. Program requirements such as 24-hour on-call coverage are not always possible. Medical record keeping, orientation of home health staff and effective and timely communication of patient care plans are more complicated. Familiarity of the patient and family with hospice staff may not be optimal.

Organizationally, the Home Care Director at Church Hospital holds a key position, as her office acts as the clearinghouse for hospice inquiries and information. Initial admission screening is accomplished through her office, as is monitoring of continuity of care and maintenance of program statistics. Working in conjunction with the hospice medical director, the Home Care Department and its corporate officer coordinate the administrative support for the program. It is important to assign day-to-day program co-ordination to a specific individual, whether it be the Home Care Director, a nursing supervisor or a person in a position created solely for this activity. Such assignment will vary according to the organizational characteristics of each program.

Further organization and implementation of the program is similar to that of other specialized patient care programs within the hospital, such as the hyperalimentation or cardiac rehabilitation program. Appropriate protocols and procedures are developed, physical facility or equipment adjustments are made, special training and orientation of personnel are conducted and interaction among members of the health care team is co-ordinated. A component not necessarily typical of specialized patient care programs is the role of the volunteer organization, headed by a director responsible for this important service.

The structure of the hospice service at Church Hospital is an example of a "program management" approach which organizationally crosses several jurisdictional lines. This is not alien to hospital operations where separate departmental functions must effectively interact in the provision of patient care. A network is designed to shift the orientation of managers away from differentiated departmental patterns and toward an integrated concept of the program into which their particular contributions must fit. In order for this approach to be successful, a concerted effort must be made to ensure that program objectives do not conflict with departmental goals and operations.

Financial Aspects

In considering the financial aspects of hospice care, most attention is given to the question of reimbursement for services. Unfortunately, this puts the cart before the horse, since little is known about the cost of hospice care, let alone reaching agreement on its legitimate components. Third party payors (most significantly the federal government and Blue Cross) are making few commitments until the cost of hospice care and its impact on the cost of health care in general are studied. Demonstration projects designed for this purpose by the federal government and Blue Cross were initiated during 1979 and 1980 throughout the United States.

The determination of costs and the financial viability of any hospice care program should begin with a look at standards of care. Acceptable standards for hospice care are of utmost concern to the public and to those committed to implementing the hospice concept without compromising its philosophy. The National Hospice Organization has labored to produce standards which are intended for use in the accreditation process (National Hospice Organization, 1979).

Since standards of care meaningfully prescribe resources necessary to characterize a program as hospice care, recognition and acceptance of minimum standards is a basic financial consideration. However, there is no present consensus on either minimal or optimal acceptable standards. The successful achievement of any standard for a contemplated or existing hospice program is in large part dependent upon its available resources. Hospitals have ready means to meet high standards in a cost effective and efficient manner through program management. Fluctuating hospice census and varying intensity of services are managed with maximum productivity through program-oriented plans and goals superimposed over existing departmental structures.

Planning

Financial analysis of hospice care is initiated in the planning process. Hospice program planning in the formal sense must identify hospice care as it relates to the organization providing the service, to those who would receive services and to political and economic realities. This is a most difficult aspect of program planning, since the product of such identification often presents the challenge of change to the system. Universal planning considerations include an analysis of need to be translated to demand and to a projected program capacity and scope. The grassroots movement from which the hospice concept developed represented a response to an unmet need. Quantification of that need is essential to organize effectively the resources required to meet it.

There is no magic formula for measuring need. Planning professionals must utilize their knowledge of the many variables involved in a given community and logically piece this data together to project an estimated demand. Planning is at best an educated guess, since the factors considered may not interact in the expected manner and important influences may not be taken into account.

Before estimates can be made, some basic definitions must be established in order to limit and identify boundaries. This may include limiting the program to cancer patients who reside within the hospital's service area.

Church Hospital employed the following method to estimate demand.

Step 1. Determine areawide hospital utilization rate: 132.4 admissions per 1,000.

Step 2. Determine the year's medical/surgical admission projection: 9,288.

Step 3. The hospital's use-rate population base therefore is:

$$\frac{9,288}{132.4} = 70.15 \times 1,000 = 70,150$$

Step 4. Approximately 50% of the hospital's admissions are from Baltimore City and about 50% are from Baltimore County and the four adjacent counties. City use-rate population base: 35,000; county use-rate population base: 35,000.

Step 5. Cancer death rates for the Baltimore area are city, 288/100,000; county, 196/100,000.

Step 6. To determine the annual number of cancer deaths from Church Hospital's use-rate population base the following computations were made: 35,000/100,000 × 288 = 98 patients from Baltimore City; 35,000/100,000 × 196 = 68.6 patients from the four counties.

Step 7. The hospital estimates, therefore, that the hospital's present market

Step 7.   share from its service area will provide approximately 170 admissions
per year to the hospice program.

This method provides a baseline number from which to work. Other factors
are subsequently analyzed and used to adjust this figure.

– Hospice care may not be appropriate or may not be desired by all patients.
– Program admission criteria such as a requirement that a caregiver be present
at home excludes some patients.
– The proportion of cancer patients in any one hospital is affected by the specialty mix of the medical staff, services available at the facility and medical
referral patterns.
– The presence or absence of other hospice care providers can make a significant impact on referrals to the program.
– It may well be determined that a specific demand exists, but that resources
are available to meet only a portion of that demand.

Once program capacity is determined, institutional costs may be calculated on
the basis of the number of beds involved and the associated overhead. Other
considerations include the need to modify existing physical facilities (e.g., add
private family lounges or redecorate rooms) and the impact of the program on
hospital census. Will patients who would otherwise be admitted to curative care
simply be reclassified as hospice patients? Will additional patients be admitted
who otherwise would receive services elsewhere or no services at all?

Every hospital will answer these questions differently. Moreover, in the face
of variables such as length of stay, physician understanding and support and the
mix of medical services provided in each hospital and its community, answers
may change over time for each hospital. Because of the financial implications of
these planning considerations, the option of developing a hospice care program
based upon a ''swing-bed'' concept and flexible use of personnel is attractive. In
this way, a developing program may still respond to community need and be
allowed to gain momentum on its own strength.

Personnel

The need for a variety of competent personnel to comprise the hospice team is a
critical cost and quality issue. The individual needs of patients and families
encompass a wide spectrum of manpower resources. A formal program structure
in a hospital setting provides the means to tap these resources for hospice care.
Otherwise, staffing may be supplemented through contractual agreements in
order to provide special services needed on an individual patient basis.

While hospice care is labor intensive, much time is contributed by volunteers.
Volunteers are essential to successful hospice care; the existence of organized

volunteer services in hospitals facilitates recruitment and involvement in the hospice care team. Through volunteer support, program staffing expenses may be defrayed. This is especially true in the context of hospice care standards, where personal attention and time to spend with the patient and family must be readily available. Special services, such as art or music therapy, may be successfully provided by volunteers.

In order for volunteer support to be financially meaningful, it must be incorporated into program planning and consistently available. Otherwise, additional staffing expense should be budgeted in order to maintain program standards. It is highly desirable, if not essential, to incur the expense of employing a volunteer director to maintain a stable and well organized volunteer component.

Home Care

Whether provided through a hospital-based department or through contract with independent agencies, home care services are integral to a hospice care program. The feasibility of hospital-based home care in general may be a major financial obstacle. Reimbursement for hospice-type home care is further complicated since visits are typically two to three times longer than other home care contacts. Bereavement follow-up, liaisons with nursing homes and the inpatient unit and other special services are not reimbursed at this time. On the other hand, co-ordination with outside home health agencies is often difficult and continuity of care issues are raised.

If a viable hospital-based home care department already exists, the prospect of increased staffing expenses must be reviewed. This includes not only the impact of the program on volume of visits and staff productivity, but the increase in administrative time needed to participate in the admission process, co-ordinate with the inpatient unit and organize other home care resources. A hospital considering the addition of a home care service should evaluate the options of providing care to hospice patients only or a combination of hospice and other patients. The differences in volume, expense, reimbursement and organizational requirements are significant, yet each is a viable alternative.

Medical Support

The expense of formal medical input varies greatly and ranges from totally volunteered services to part- and full-time compensation for physician services. Unless key physicians understand, support and actively participate in its development, a hospice care program will never get off the ground. Major educational efforts must be made with the medical staff in general and with individuals on a physician-to-physician basis. At least one physician is needed to actively participate in program management, medical policy development, screening and acceptance of patients and consultative services.

The method of reimbursement for physicians' services is influenced by the particular organizational structure of a program and its setting. In a program where patients are transferred to the care of a hospice physician, fee-for-service reimbursement through billing of third party payors is possible. However, reimbursement for physician visits to the home is not sufficient to encourage this service. In any event, such compensation does not cover physicians' services on an administrative level. Administrative overhead is further increased when the hospice physician acts as program consultant to the attending physician who continues to care for his patient. Depending on the nature of services and the average time involved, reimbursement for medico-administrative services may take the form of a flat fee payable on a monthly basis. A salaried position is also an option for compensation. In a hospital where a salaried physician already plays a medico-administrative role, it may be possible to include hospice care as one of his responsibilities.

Reimbursement

Once the projected expense of a hospice program is calculated, that expense may then be related to the reimbursement system. Funds received from grants, endowments or other special trust sources are useful in underwriting start-up expenses, but generally cannot be relied upon for continued operational support on a large scale. The resources of self-paying patients are often sorely taxed by the costs of prolonged illness and/or the aggressive curative treatment which usually precedes hospice care. As with other forms of health care, third party reimbursement in the form of Medicare, state medical assistance and commercial insurance comprises the major source of operating funds.

Since this reimbursement system categorizes health care services according to levels, hospice care is reimbursed according to services approved under acute (hospital), intermediate (nursing home) or home care levels. These three categories offer a simplistic description of levels of care; a confusing and lengthy terminology exists which describes levels of care from regulatory and medical viewpoints. It is not difficult to see how official reimbursement definitions and policies shape and influence the nature of health care services delivery. A program such as hospice care does not fit the mold. Paradoxically, hospice care takes issue with the reimbursement system while simultaneously courting its support.

Hospice care is not recognized as a separate category of provider care. The continuity of care embraced by the hospice concept is disrupted by the reimbursement system, which strictly defines the circumstances and services for payment (i.e., conditions of participation). Third party reimbursement at the skilled nursing home and intermediate levels of care is generally not sufficient to cover the labor intensive expense of hospice patients. However, major components of hospice care do fall within reimbursement guidelines and provide a foundation for the survival of a program. In the acute level, virtually all services are covered by third parties. Much less coverage is available for home care and reimbursement guidelines are particularly restrictive in the hospice context. Usually absent is third party reimbursement for program components such as bereavement followup, respite care, art therapy and many professional consultative services. Nonetheless, payment for basic home care service is widely available, although not always chosen by the consumer, including employers, when purchasing insurance coverage.

The aforementioned conditions of participation serve to monitor and control utilization as a safeguard for limited resources. Such guidelines are designed to combat fraud and abuse of the reimbursement system and to contain costs. Examples of requirements and exclusions that present problems to hospice care include:

– The requirement that, to be eligible for home care or skilled nursing facility services, the patient must have been hospitalized for at least 3 days prior to admission to the lower level of care.
– The requirement that, to be eligible for home care services, the patient must be homebound; that is, unable to leave home except for infrequent or brief absences to obtain services in another setting.
– The exclusion of drugs and biologicals provided in the home and self-administered.
– The exclusion of reimbursement for bereavement counseling to the family by a nurse or other qualified professional after the death of a hospice patient.
– Restrictions on reimbursement for visits made by the hospice team to hospice patients who have been reinstitutionalized.

It is against this background that a hospice program faces a now-too-familiar financial dilemma. Given the calculated expense of a program and current reimbursement policy, a plan to handle resulting deficits must be developed. The nature and extent of deficits will vary according to the circumstances of a particular program. Several avenues may be pursued; they include:

1. An increase in the degree of volunteer support.
2. The ability of the hospital to increase general overhead expenses to be justifiably allocated to other cost centers.
3. The possibility of co-ordinating liaisons with other agencies, health care providers or private groups.
4. Special funding or grant monies.

In the long run, if gaps in reimbursement are to be filled or special legislation passed to provide for hospice care, it must be shown that a savings to the health care system is possible and/or that other benefits outweigh the expense. Several reimbursement guidelines themselves serve as barriers to the cost containment opportunities offered by hospice care. The requirement for a new plan of treatment upon a patient's discharge following reinstitutionalization creates unnecessary administrative expense; other requirements tying reimbursement to episodes of illness in acute care facilities force patients into the most expensive setting, while those exclusions denying reimbursement for certain skilled and non-skilled supportive services restrict preventive health care measures.

The savings potential of hospice care is primarily a matter of providing an alternative to expensive acute care technology. It is unlikely that savings achieved from the preventive care aspects of hospice care can be quantified. Cost containment opportunities do exist in the avoidance of an acute level of care and, when hospitalization is indicated, in less expensive palliative treatment. Just how much less is the object of much speculation.

Breindel and Gravely's (1980) study of Church Hospital's experience has shown that the total direct labor cost per patient day for the hospice patient is less than for the average medical-surgical patient. While this finding is surprising, it is not unusual to find that hospice patients utilize ancillary services to a much lesser extent than the average medical-surgical patient. Breindel found that the average charge per patient day was 27% less than the average charge per patient day hospital-wide and 50% less than the average charge per patient day when compared with other terminal patients with the same length of stay. Savings are more significant if one assumes that the alternative for many terminally ill cancer patients is an intensive battery of expensive curative measures more costly than those used by the average patient. A comparison of costs with comparable medical-surgical patients is shown on Table 1.

These findings accentuate the need for valid statistical measures, in-depth program evaluation and accurate financial analyses to enhance reimbursement prospects for hospice care. While it is encouraging to find evidence of cost efficiency, it is of little value unless the program meets its objectives and standards.

Staffing

The heart of a hospice care program is its staffing. Proper staffing of the program allows it to realize its stated objectives, not only through the numbers of individuals involved and their professional credentials, but through their special commitment to the hospice concept. Staffing is also the heart of the expense of hospice care and should be analyzed to measure resources needed for the program and to compare its cost to other forms of health care.

Table I. Comparison of Average Costs of Hospice and Comparable Medical-Surgical Patients (Breindel and Gravely, 1980).

	Hospice Patient	Medical-Surgical Patient
Room	$1,547.58	$1,784.02
Pharmacy	$ 58.77	$ 294.60
Laboratory	$ 24.82	$ 405.12
Radiology	$ 29.89	$ 265.91
Respiratory Therapy	$ 77.40	$ 73.07
Admission	$ 73.45	$ 73.45
Supplies	$ 64.97	$ 95.95
Electrocardiography	$ 8.41	$ 57.69
Physical Therapy	$ 9.38	$ 30.14
Other	$ 26.27	$ 351.36
Charge Per Patient Day	$ 173.94	$ 345.30
Charge Per Admission	$1,920.84	$3,431.35

Cost Accounting

Due to the nature of program integration at Church Hospital, it is difficult to segregate the expense of staffing for hospice care. No separate "cost center" exists to isolate costs; staff participate in the care of other patients and their activities in hospice care vary with hospice census and the individual needs of patients in the program. While program responsiveness and productivity are enhanced by the integrated structure, this advantage is lost if hospice-related expense is not monitored. The depth of professional disciplines and numbers of personnel are of no use to the program if other responsibilities conflict with hospice care. Consequently, program capacity and, therefore, expense is directly related to the staffing needs of hospice patients.

In order to identify staffing expense, a study was undertaken using management engineering techniques to determine the time spent in providing care by each discipline (Breindel and Gravely, 1980). In a comparison with staffing required by the average medical/surgical patient at the hospital, it was found that the hospice patient received less nursing care from the nursing staff than a medical/surgical patient (3.9 hours per patient day, as compared to 4.4 hours per patient day). However, when nursing care supplemented *by volunteers and family* was taken into account, total time spent in nursing activities was 7.3 hours per patient day. This finding underscores the role of volunteers and the general interaction with the family in maintaining a high standard of hospice care.

Other disciplines were found to spend more time with the hospice patient than with the average medical/surgical patient. They include physical therapists, dietitians, nurse practitioners, social workers and others. However, due to the "savings" in nursing time provided by volunteers and family, total labor cost per patient day for the hospice patient was less than for the average medical/surgical patient. The alternative of staff designated solely for hospice care presumes a caseload consistently large enough to justify the expense. This may be realistic for certain core personnel such as nurses and social workers, but becomes less certain for other professionals, such as physical therapists, dietitians or respiratory therapists. Here it can be seen that the relationship between available resources, program standards and estimated patient volume significantly impacts upon the proper mix of employees, volunteers and contracted services which comprise program staffing.

Program Integration and the Hospice Team

The integration of hospice patients into a general medical/surgical unit and into the total workload of each hospice team member was intended for more than cost efficiency. Its aim was also to alleviate staff stress associated with caring for the terminally ill. This integration also aids in alleviating the pressure associated with participating in what is perceived to be a novel and pioneering program. Subjective feedback from staff at Church Hospital supports this approach.

A staffing consideration of special importance in an integrated program such as Church Hospital's is the establishment of the hospice team concept. Without the unifying force of active teamwork, co-ordination would break down, continuity would be lost and personal stress would be magnified. Any cost efficiencies achieved would be impossible without the team effort; integration of volunteers into the working nursing unit and into the home care field is a prime example of this.

In order to have an effective hospice team, staffing should include a variety of professional disciplines to provide depth and expertise. Hospitals have excellent access to health care professions and the means to orient and incorporate them into the hospice care team.

The Church Hospital team includes home care nursing, inpatient nursing, social workers, chaplains, physical therapists, dieticians, volunteers, nurse practitioners and physicians. Support is provided from the pharmacy, respiratory therapy and all other hospital departments. Psychiatric services and other specialized personnel are available and ready to respond to an individual patient's need. Chapter 6 describes the components and co-ordination of the hospice team in the clinical setting.

Continuity of Care

The hospice concept strives to eliminate the fragmented health care which occurs when patients move from one delivery setting to another. Staffing patterns and responsibilities can be utilized to achieve optimal coordination of patient care plans and maintain familiar and secure relationships with the patient and family. At Church Hospital, key personnel who act to insure continuity of care include home health nursing, the chaplain, the social worker, volunteers and the hospice physicians. This function is well understood by the staff involved and is an essential thread tying the program together and influencing interaction with other personnel. Patient rounds are alternated with team conferences on a weekly basis as an additional mechanism to insure co-ordination and optimal patient care.

In a hospital-based program providing inpatient and home care services, continuity is jeopardized if the patient for some reason cannot be at home when he does not require acute care. This circumstance is controlled for the most part by admission screening criteria, but cannot be avoided entirely. In the absence of affiliation with a skilled nursing home or intermediate care provider, hospice staff ordinarily maintain some continuity of care through volunteer efforts. The concept of *continuity visits* by hospice staff as a reimbursable service is being considered by some third party payors, but is not now a reality. Those patients who are not eligible for admission to a particular program due to the absence of a caregiver in the home are of concern to all hospice programs. In most states the free-standing hospice is not recognized as a provider category and it appears that staffing requirements present a major deterrent to the nursing home industry in developing hospice care.

References

Breindel, C.L. and Gravely, G.E.: *Costs of Providing a Mixed-Unit Hospice Program.* Working paper. Dept. of Health Administration, Medical College of Virginia. (1980)

National Hospice Organization: *Standards of a Hospice Program of Care.* (1979)

9. Questions Most Commonly Asked About Hospice Care

As we have spoken with individuals and groups about our work in the care of the terminally ill, certain questions recur frequently. Some of these questions help to crystallize issues and problems. Others permit a different focus on some of the complex matters covered elsewhere in this text. For these reasons, it seems useful to deal directly with these questions here.

Questions Regarding Hospice Care in General

Is there a means by which hospices are certified or approved?

The name "hospice" has been used by various institutions for centuries and is still in use today by institutions which have little or nothing to do with the care of the terminally ill. In most places there is, as yet, no restriction on the use of this term.

There is unquestionably a need for the development of standards for hospice care of the terminally ill and some means by which hospice programs for the care of the terminally ill can be certified or approved. At present, such a mechanism does not exist, but the National Hospice Organization (NHO) is giving this matter high priority. NHO has been formed by the leaders of hospice care in America and is in the process of establishing standards of hospice care. Once standards are agreed upon, a mechanism for survey of individual programs will have to be established. It is the fervent hope of many of us involved in hospice care that standards will be set and accreditation provided by caregivers rather than by government agencies.

No one can question the desirability of establishing criteria of adequate hospice care and of developing an accreditation mechanism. This is needed to prevent abuse of the hospice approach and the development of substandard programs. It is also necessary in order to permit programs to be reimbursed through health insurance plans. However, we must remember that hospice care is a dynamic field and that there is still a great deal to learn. Innovation must be encouraged. Standards, therefore, must allow sufficient flexibility to permit progress and avoid stagnation.

Hospice care is really not new, is it? Isn't it just a
return to old values and approaches?

In some measure it is correct that hospice includes a return to traditional values and methods. It re-establishes the kind of personal concern and attention which we associate with a bygone era; this personal concern has decreased in many aspects of modern medical care, particularly in dealing with the dying. Much of the value of hospice care derives from its re-emphasis on the traditions of caring, which have been such an integral part of the medical and nursing professions.

However, there are some features of hospice care that are relatively new; they present an opportunity to apply modern techniques and approaches to the old traditions. The multidisciplinary nature of hospice care is an example; it applies, in co-ordinated fashion, the technology of *many* trained and skilled professionals. Certain specifics of patient care are also relatively new. From the work of Twycross (1974) and others we have learned a great deal about pain control in the terminally ill. The technique described for managing intestinal obstruction in advanced malignancy without the use of nasogastric tubes and intravenous solutions represents a departure from conventional care. It utilizes drugs such as stool softeners and anti-emetics, which were not available before the era of nasogastric tubes and intravenous fluids.

In a sense, hospice care permits us to return to useful old values and techniques but with a much improved prospect for effectiveness.

Won't hospice care lead to the development of one more specialty
and thus further fragmentation in medicine?

It is too early to tell at this point to what extent hospice care will establish itself as a specialty. It certainly is an area in which some workers will concentrate their interest. To the extent that the terminally ill profit from this specialization, the benefits in care outweigh the disadvantages of fragmentation. Unquestionably, the development of anesthesiology as a specialty further fragmented medicine, but few of us would want to be put to sleep with an unskilled person administering our anesthetic.

In a very real sense, hospice care is holistic; one of its aims is to bring to bear on the patient and his family, in a co-ordinated fashion, the benefits of many disciplines. It may thus teach us something about how to deal with fragmentation in other areas of medical care.

*Isn't there a risk that patients with potentially curable cancer will
be regarded as hopelessly ill and entered in a hospice care program?*

In a patient with malignant disease, the decision that the patient's condition is incurable must *always* be made cautiously and carefully. The existence of hospice care does not change this imperative.

Sometimes it is easily evident that a malignant tumor is beyond the point of cure. On other occasions it may be very difficult to make a decision. In such circumstances the availability of hospice care may in actuality make it easier to crystallize this decision. It is usually much more satisfactory to make a clear choice rather than to evade the issue.

With hospice care as an option, it becomes somewhat simpler to face the decision more forthrightly. Presently there is sometimes a tendency to continue invasive, uncomfortable therapeutic measures directed against an incurable tumor simply because there is nothing else to do.

In those instances in which there is doubt about whether or not there is a reasonable chance for cure, the use of ample consultation and Tumor Board consideration can be valuable. Both the physician making referral to a hospice care program and the physicians operating the program must be certain that the available evidence indicates that further efforts at cure of the disease do not have a reasonable prospect of success.

We feel that it is extremely important that management of the terminally ill through hospice care be a part of the continuum of medical care, rather than something outside the remainder of the health care system. This is necessary, in part, because of this type of issue at the curative-palliative interface.

The rapid developments in the treatment of certain forms of malignant disease make it essential that hospice physicians remain informed about advances in oncology. Rarely, new treatment methods may convert a previously incurable patient into one who can be cured; such a patient should promptly be placed upon appropriate therapy for his disease. In short, hospice care does not mean that any patient with a reasonable chance of cure will be deprived of that chance.

Isn't hospice care really a form of euthanasia?

Definitely not, by almost any accepted definition of euthanasia. On the contrary, the aim of hospice care is, in a sense, to make euthanasia *irrelevant* for those who are terminally ill from malignant disease. Its goal is to make death as painless as possible. To the extent that dying is gentler and more comfortable, the issue of hastening death becomes less relevant.

We would be less than candid, though, if we did not say that the issue of providing palliation to the terminally ill must be looked at in two dimensions, both in terms of quantity of life and quality of life. The over-riding objective in dealing with the terminally ill is to stretch life in *both* dimensions. However, hospice care is committed to the principle that in those instances where a choice must be made between making living more comfortable and extending life, the only rational decision is to do everything possible to improve the quality of life. Experience with hospice care suggests that this is a choice that very seldom has to be made.

One might also inquire whether the administration of relatively high doses of potent narcotics shortens life. This is unlikely since these drugs are administered in such a fashion as to adjust the dose carefully to keep the patient not only quite conscious but actually alert.

There is no evidence to suggest that patients in a hospice care program have a shorter life expectancy than similar patients treated outside of a hospice care program. We have some reason to suspect, in fact, that through the relief of symptoms life in actuality is prolonged for some patients. Perhaps this occurs through that nebulous but very real "will to live."

How do you get physician support for developing a hospice program?

This question, which is usually asked by non-physicians who are familiar with hospice concepts and wish to start a program in their community, recognizes the critical importance of physician support for such a program. It is virtually impossible to undertake any type of meaningful hospice care without the endorsement and involvement of physicians. It is futile to consider generating a hospital-based program without the active participation of the hospital medical staff.

To a large extent the answer to this question depends upon local factors and perhaps upon some intangibles. There is no substitute for the "right chemistry." We think, however, that certain measures are of great help. The first is identifying and enlisting the enthusiastic involvement of certain key physicians. Within the organization of any medical community, there are identifiable physicians who have a great deal of influence with their colleagues. From among these it is usually possible to interest and enlist several who will serve as catalysts.

It is important to recognize that physician involvement must occur *early* in the planning stages. Nothing discourages physician participation faster than to be presented with a virtually fully developed protocol for a program that has been developed without physician input. As soon as the key physicians are sufficiently familiar with hospice care, they should begin to involve other physicians in planning.

From the first, physicians must see hospice care as a *tool* to use in the care of their patients, not as a threat that will limit their therapeutic options, steal their patients or tangle them in paperwork. This requires very careful description of exactly what problems hospice care solves and the ways in which it does so. Factual presentation, not evangelism, convinces physicians.

In securing physician support, the option for the attending physician either to continue in the care of the patient or to turn the patient over to the hospice physician was most helpful. In this way hospice care was seen by a large number of physicians as something they could use to solve problems.

Finally, patience and perseverance are important. Physicians are besieged with new techniques that are purported to offer advantages and benefits. They have learned, for their own defense and that of their patients, to be skeptical about such proposals and to be cautious in their acceptance. More than we realize, all of us are the beneficiaries of this attitude.

The most effective means of securing physician support is to demonstrate repeatedly what hospice care will do for their patients. A few physicians will remain unconvinced until the experience is first hand. Some of the most skeptical doubters on our medical staff became avid supporters of the program once it was in operation. We, incidently, owe a special debt to these physicians, for we learned much from their doubts.

What about malpractice suits in hospice programs?

Hospice care apparently has rarely led to malpractice suits; even more rare is a suit in which the plaintiff has been successful. Although the author has not made an exhaustive study of this topic, at this writing he does not know of a judgment rendered against a hospice caregiver arising directly out of hospice care.

In the United States today, there are growing numbers of civil suits for damages in most fields. The paucity of such suits in England where hospice care has been in operation for longer is little comfort, because the ground rules in both legal matters (where there is no contingency fee) and in a national health system of medical care are strikingly different.

Furthermore, hospice care is in a sense at high risk because it literally deals with life and death situations, with emotion-charged issues and with a circumstance in which ''failure'' is the normal outcome. The decision to undertake no further curative therapy and the delegation of responsibilities to volunteers and families unquestionably raise the medico-legal vulnerability of hospice workers. The existence of extended family, not all of whom may be identified during the terminal illness, raises some special problems.

Nonetheless, it is not surprising that malpractice suits have been a very uncommon experience for hospices. There is a great deal of evidence to suggest that a common denominator among a vast majority of malpractice actions is the lack of the very things that hospice care emphasizes: strong interpersonal relationships, deep sympathetic concern and meaningful communication.

What has been the reaction to your program?

The reaction has been overwhelmingly favorable. It has been seen on the faces of, and heard in the words of, innumerable patients. It has been described in touching fashion by bereaved loved ones. Almost without exception, the medical staff of the hospital, as individuals and as a group, have given their enthusiastic endorsement. Interest in the community has been substantial and is reflected in the initiation of other programs. Third party payors and government agencies have reacted favorably in a number of ways. We have made no formal effort to measure and document reaction in these various groups and feel that efforts to do so would only prove the obvious.

What are the major problems your hospice faces today?

This is a question which doubtless would be answered somewhat differently by different members of our hospice care team. The following is the author's response and thus represents the perspective of the chairman of the hospice care committee.

Reimbursement for services is incomplete; it is thus difficult to make the program pay for itself. Most inpatient reimbursement formulae have been as satisfactory for hospice as for non-hospice patients, but better means need to be found to cover outpatient expenses. As always, finances are of critical importance, but the better reimbursement for inpatient as compared to outpatient care presents some special impediments to ideal care for the terminally ill.

Work load and staff assignments require study and modification. Breindel and Gravely's work (1980) has begun to provide some data that can be used for this purpose. As more members of our medical staff become familiar with the principles of hospice care, we hope that more of them will serve as attending physician for patients in the program and thus lighten the demands upon the hospice physician. Training of additional volunteers for evening and night duty would be helpful. In some measure, there is a question of properly distributing personnel to meet the demands; we have not had the information to permit doing this in a rational way. For reasons evident from Breindel and Gravely's study, much of the frustration that personnel in the program experience is not specifically related to hospice care, but simply to the work load on the nursing unit to which hospice patients are assigned.

There is need for additional educational programs both for hospice personnel and for others whose work has an impact on the hospice program. Medical staff members who refer patients need a clearer perception of what the program offers. Members of the medical staff who serve as attending physicians for their patients in the program need continuing education in principles of hospice care. Nursing personnel and volunteers need continuing education as well.

In order for us to learn as much as possible from our growing experience, improved methods of data collection and analysis are needed. Through this we will learn by doing and others can profit from our experience.

Our limited ability to deal effectively with certain symptoms, such as anorexia and weakness, is a source of frustration and dissatisfaction. We hope that clinical experience, properly investigated, will lead to some breakthroughs.

Won't the development of a cure for cancer make hospices obsolete?

Unfortunately, we are unlikely to see for some time that happy day when there is a uniformly effective method of prevention or treatment for cancer. Meanwhile, hospice care can accomplish an immense amount of good and can have a favorable impact on medical care in general. Even when cancer is no longer a threat, there will doubtless be other diseases for which the application of hospice principles and practice will be useful.

Questions Regarding a Hospital-Based Hospice Program

What are the advantages of a hospital-based program?

This question is difficult to answer briefly because it involves a number of complex issues. To list them is cumbersome. Nonetheless, there are several points worth making.

A hospital-based or affiliated program can be developed within the framework of the present health care system in most communities. This has a number of very important advantages.

The transition from curative to palliative care often is easier if it does not require the patient to make an adjustment to a totally new setting or personnel. Since many patients enter a hospice program as inpatients, this is a particularly important consideration.

Similarly, once in a hospice program the ease of access to more sophisticated forms of treatment may be an important factor in determining whether or not such measures are used. It is often argued that hospice care by its nature does not require much technological support. This is true, but we have found that circumstances do occur in which the ready access to facilities located in the hospital has been extremely helpful in providing palliation. This applies not just to antitumor therapy such as surgery, radiation and chemotherapy, but also to other support measures such as intra-medullary nailing to prevent pathologic fractures and tracheotomy for upper airway obstruction. We feel that the ready availability of the entire spectrum of care that a hospital offers has improved the caliber of palliative care which we can offer.

Communications between those providing day-by-day hospice care and others who might contribute to the comfort of the patient are simpler and more effective in the hospital setting. For a patient with vertebral metastases from breast carcinoma who shows signs of impending paraplegia, on-the-spot consultation with the neurosurgeon, oncologist and radiotherapist can be of inestimable value.

The most common criticism of hospital-based hospice programs has to do with the impersonal, inflexible and frightening environment of the hospital and its institutional policies. It is said that only outside of a hospital can an environment be created in which patients can be comfortable and relaxed. Our experience indicates that this is simply not so. We make no pretense to being able to provide all of the comforts of home in our hospital, but then neither does any type of institution, hospital or free-standing hospice. This is why we all believe so strongly in home care. Nonetheless, we have found it possible to create within the hospital a very suitable atmosphere for the proper rendering of hospice care. It is feasible to relax hospital regulations for hospice care patients sufficiently to permit comfort in a degree comparable to that achievable in any institutional setting.

In looking at free-standing and hospital-based programs, we prefer not to take an either/or approach. At this point, either may be the preferable—or the only possible—place to begin, depending upon local circumstances. Neither can be regarded as totally meeting the needs of the terminally ill patient. The hospital-based program with home care is handicapped in handling the patient who does not require hospital care but whose home circumstances do not permit management there. The free-standing unit with home care is limited in its ability to handle the patient who would profit from inhospital care. Both types of units must strive to develop methods that permit them to cover the entirety of the spectrum of care needed by terminally ill patients.

*Even in a hospital-based program, wouldn't it be better
to have a separate unit for hospice patients?*

This question can probably best be dealt with by looking at two aspects of the design of inhospital hospice facilities. The first is patient care. There are no controlled studies to tell us whether patients are better handled in a separate unit or when integrated with other hospital patients. We *can* say that the interaction between hospice and non-hospice patients on the nursing unit which houses our hospice patients has usually been positive in both directions. More frequently than not, hospice and non-hospice patients have each had a beneficial effect upon the other. There have been very few problems related to this arrangement. Furthermore, by not having a separate unit for hospice patients, our staff has been involved with both hospice and general medical-surgical patients. This has avoided some of the psychological problems for personnel who are handling only terminally ill patients experienced by many hospice programs. It has also permitted some of the desirable features of hospice care to cross-fertilize general medical care in a way that would otherwise not have been possible.

The other consideration is of course the matter of economics. The establishment of a separate facility, whether it is some place outside the hospital, on a specially designated floor of the hospital, or at the end of a corridor, necessitates some construction costs. But this is not the most important consideration. What is of critical importance, particularly for the medium-sized or small hospital, is flexibility in bed usage. To the extent that beds are set aside for specific purposes, a hospital's ability to utilize the total number of its existing beds is diminished. Since, in one 3-month period, we experienced a variation of daily inpatient hospice census from one to twelve patients, it is easy to see the impact that designated beds or a separate unit would have. Using a "swing bed" system such as that at Church Hospital probably makes having a hospice program feasible for many hospitals for which it would otherwise not be practical.

In summary, if those of us who have been involved in the hospice program at Church Hospital were offered the opportunity to have a separate unit for our patients, there would probably be split opinion. We would be unanimous, however, in our response to the question of whether we would rather have a hospice program with swing beds or no program at all.

Aside from a separate unit and swing beds on a general unit, what other organizational options are there for a hospital-based hospice program?

So-called "scatter beds" may be used throughout the hospital. This approach has been employed with fair success by a number of programs. Its disadvantages are related to the dispersion of patients to widely separated areas throughout the hospital. This usually requires that the hospice team be a consultative service—a symptom support control team. Such an arrangement, although apparently the best approach under certain circumstances, lacks the cohesive impact of a hospice team functioning in a specific nursing unit with the option for the hospice physician to serve as the attending physician for some of the patients in the program.

What has been the attitude of other patients toward the hospice program?

On all general medical-surgical nursing units with semi-private rooms, patients have been exposed to the terminally ill, so that this has presented no particular problem. Naturally, one of our initial concerns was whether non-hospice patients would resent the relaxation of hospital regulations for hospice patients. This simply has not been a problem; on the few occasions on which questions have been raised, brief explanations by the staff have been well accepted. The two way interaction between hospice and non-hospice patients has often been profitable for each.

What has been the effect of the hospice program on the care of other patients?

At this point we have no data on this topic, only impressions. There is some reason to believe that the re-emphasis of some of the traditional values of medical care, including the meaningful communication and sympathetic concern which are such an important part of hospice care, have rubbed off onto the care provided non-hospice patients. The question might be raised whether the increased demand for personal attention to hospice patients on the part of staff might not diminish the attention directed to non-hospice patients on the same unit. This does not seem to happen.

Breindel and Gravely's data (1980) indicate that, although hospice patients take more total personnel time than non-hospice patients, this increased time is given largely by volunteers and family. This suggests an explanation for the observation that decreased attention to non-hospice patients has not occurred.

Questions Regarding Organization and Financing of a Hospice Program

How expensive is hospice care?

Among those who have observed hospice programs, there is no doubt that it is "care effective." Determining whether or not it is "cost effective" is a complicated matter. It may be an impossible task, since no one can find a means of placing a dollar value on human comfort.

In addressing this question, one must also take a look at the basis of comparison. If hospice care is compared to conscientious conventional treatment for the terminally ill, including prolonged hospitalization, numerous diagnostic tests and the liberal use of radiation and chemotherapy, hospice care is almost certainly more economical. On the other hand, if hospice care is compared to virtually no care at all, it is clearly more expensive.

At this point there are no data that permit reasonable comparison of the management of terminal illness in conventional fashion and in a hospice care program. The following may be of some help, however.

For inpatients, hospice care is clearly labor intensive. Although it is a relatively low level of care technologically, with far fewer diagnostic and therapeutic maneuvers, it does require a high level of personal attention. A substantial portion of this attention, however, can be provided by volunteers and by family once they have gained a certain level of understanding. Breindel and Gravely's data (1980) compare hospice patients with intermediate care general medical-surgical patients, the vast majority of whom are not terminally ill. Those data indicate that the average cost per patient day for hospice patients is approximately one-half that of non-hospice patients.

In addition, it is reasonable to presume that hospice care permits a far larger percentage of the terminal illness to be spent as an outpatient than would be possible under conventional care. Thus, hospital stays are shorter. On the other hand, outpatient care costs are doubtless higher for hospice than for non-hospice patients.

The bottom line would seem to be that, when somewhat lower daily inpatient costs and shorter hospital stays are combined with somewhat higher outpatient costs, hospice care offers an economically attractive alternative to traditional terminal care.

How do you get reimbursed for hospice care?

For inpatients, reimbursement is the same as for non-hospice inpatients. Hospice patients who require hospitalization would require it whether or not they were in a hospice program. As a consequence, third party payors use the same rules as they would for any other hospitalized patient.

Reimbursement for outpatient care is a more complex matter. Some patients possess home care coverage as part of their health insurance; for these, many services are reimbursed. For patients who do not have a home care provision in their health insurance, there is little or no reimbursement from third party carriers. In such instances the patient is billed; any balance beyond what the patient can pay has to be secured from other sources such as grants and donations. To the extent that it cannot be recovered, it must be accepted as a loss.

But even for patients who possess insurance that covers home care, certain features of such coverage are often not suitable for hospice care. There are often stipulations, for example, that there must have been a prior period of hospitalization or that the patient be homebound. These are requirements which many hospice patients do not meet; as a consequence, home care service for them is not reimbursed. Furthermore, home care visits for hospice patients are usually longer than are those for patients on other types of home care. Since reimbursement formulae do not take this into account, the provider of care is not fully compensated.

It is in the area of coverage for outpatients, then, that there is the greatest need for improvement. This, incidentally, is a problem not confined to hospice programs. By and large, insurance carriers are offering increasing options for various types of home care coverage. There is need for a larger number of such policies covering more services. However, it is the purchasers of policies who will determine whether or not such options sell. Individuals and groups such as companies and labor unions need to be educated in the value of having insurance which will cover home care services.

Bereavement and other counseling services present a special problem. It is difficult to imagine that in the foreseeable future such services will be covered by any type of health insurance. Other options must be found for financing this aspect of hospice care.

Have you added staff to the nursing unit that houses the hospice inpatients?

Little if any change was made in the staffing pattern on the 50-bed general medical-surgical unit when we began housing all hospice patients there. Study of nursing time per patient (Breindel and Gravely, 1980) suggests that the overall staffing requirements are not greatly altered by having hospice patients on a nursing unit. Although more total personnel time is required in the management of hospice than of non-hospice patients, this difference is largely made up by volunteers and family. Thus, except for the addition of volunteers, there has been little need to change the total number of personnel assigned to the unit. What has taken place is some change in the individuals making up the staff. Some of the staff assigned to that nursing unit did not wish to be involved in hospice care and some employees on other units requested assignment to the hospice floor. As far as possible, these requests for changes have been honored.

What problems have you had with staff stress and burn out and what do you do about it?

Probably because personnel on the nursing unit containing hospice patients deal with both hospice and non-hospice patients, we have had few of the problems that arise from day-to-day exposure exclusively to the dying. As noted above, some staff members have found themselves unsuited to the care of the terminally ill; since this nursing unit has a disproportionate percentage of patients in this category, they have requested transfer to other units. Usually it has been the staff member himself who has first recognized the desirability of transfer.

What almost every member of our staff has experienced in some degree is the common syndrome of overwork. In his 30 years in medicine, the author has not found a totally satisfactory solution to this problem. This is partly due to the fact that some of the satisfactions of taking care of patients are deeply intertwined with factors that lead to overwork.

General problems related to the work load have unquestionably been aggravated occasionally by specific difficulties related to providing care to the terminally ill. Fears regarding one's own death, grief over a patient to whom one has felt particularly close, and insecurity about one's role in the multidisciplinary team do occur.

We have not developed a formal structured system for dealing with staff stress. Although each member of the hospice team has doubtless at some time been very important to other members in coping with stress-related problems, the intimate involvement of our chaplains in the program has made them a particularly valuable resource in dealing with stress. At the biweekly patient conference, staff members are encouraged to express any specific personal concerns or difficulties they may have had with the patients under discussion. This has often led to helpful sharing in the group.

The section on Staff Stress in Chapter 6 addresses this issue more systematically and in more detail.

Questions Regarding Patient Care in a Hospice Program

How are patients selected for the program?

The program is designed for patients of members of our medical staff who are terminally ill from malignant disease. Some patients who are not under the care of the Church Hospital medical staff are accepted.

Any attending physician who has a patient whom he feels is suitable for entry into the program makes a referral to the hospice program. If the patient meets the guidelines described in Chapter 2, he is accepted. On occasion, the work load in the program is such that no additional patients can be accommodated, in which case an accepted patient is placed on a priority list in accordance with the severity of symptom control problems he presents.

What are patients in the program told about their disease?

This question is difficult to answer both well and briefly. It could be the subject of a book itself. There are many ramifications and much need for individualization. A few points are, however, worth making.

The first thing one must understand is that in dealing with the patient dying of advanced malignancy it is much more important to *listen* than to tell. It is only when one perceives what the patient presently knows, wishes to know and needs to know that one can provide meaningful help. One must listen carefully to what the patient tells; one must be sensitive to non-verbal language and to the real meaning of questions, as well as to questions not asked. Nothing worthwhile can be conveyed to a patient in a speech or lecture about his condition; genuine dialogue is essential.

On the one hand, most patients with advanced malignancy strongly suspect or really "know" what their situation is. It is difficult to be even mildly ill these days without imagining that one has incurable malignancy. Patients with cancer bring to their illness a background of awareness about malignancy and are usually quite sensitive to the verbal and other signals being sent by those around them.

On the other hand, almost every patient experiences denial in some degree whenever he first perceives that he has an incurable disease. This denial must be appraised with respect to its intensity and its value as a defense mechanism. It must then be taken into consideration as one approaches the matter of discussing with the patient his understanding of his situation.

For those patients who know, or almost know, the true situation, there are many benefits to be derived from having it confirmed in the right way at the right time. Often unpleasant truth is easier to bear than uncertainty. The truth opens avenues that permit the patient to talk about and be reassured on those points that may be of concern to him. For example, he can bring out his fears about pain and death; this, in turn, makes it possible to deal with these fears. He can speak with his loved ones about the things most important to them. He can cope with practical problems such as finances in a much more prudent fashion.

It seems to me to be a hoax of the cruelest and most absurd dimensions to refuse to discuss with a patient who already understands his situation the facts that he wants and needs to know. By listening carefully one can determine what the patient suspects, what he would like confirmed and what additional information he needs to have. In addition to listening, it is important to provide the information with kindly candor, telling the truth within the patient's ability to understand.

It is important to recognize that you can not tell a person something he refuses to know. Attempting to convey the truth to a patient who is not ready to accept that he is dying is futile. For patients who are not ready—and some are never ready, even at the moment of death—it is pointless and probably harmful to enter into vigorous efforts to get through to them.

What I have said so far is fine as a generalization, but if any matter requires individualization it is this. There is an immense individuality in patients' capacity to know and understand their disease and its implications. Sensitivity of the highest order is required to detect a particular patient's readiness to talk. In addition, this readiness is not a static thing; it will change in either direction from day to day.

Two final comments on this matter of the patient's understanding of his status should be made. First, the almost moment by moment variation in *acceptance* should be emphasized. This can be quite striking in some patients and is distinct from the patient's variable readiness to talk. It is not uncommon to have a patient, almost in sequence, discuss his impending death and describe plans for something 4 or 5 years in the future. The other point is to remember to be non-judgmental with respect to the patient's level of understanding of his status. Many of us have an instinctive inclination to feel that the most realistic appraisal is the best. In truth, for some patients, denial to the bitter end may be the best of all options.

What are the common problems that necessitate hospitalization of hospice patients?

The basic rule, of course, is that it is generally better to manage the patient at home if this can be done. Hospitalization, however, can be necessitated by a number of problems.

Many of our patients are in the hospital when they enter the program. The fact that they have terminal malignancy and are candidates for hospice care has been discovered while the patient is hospitalized. As soon as such patients can be managed at home, they are discharged from the hospital.

The single most common reason for admission to inpatient status is probably inadequate pain control. Although patients can be managed on very high doses of narcotic at home, the titration process by which the optimal pattern of narcotic administration is achieved requires close observation and frequent dosage changes which are difficult to execute outside the hospital.

Mental confusion often necessitates hospitalization. No matter what the home situation, it can be very difficult to manage a confused, restless, agitated patient at home.

Severe insomnia poses difficult problems for the caregivers at home. An uncomfortable, sleepless patient saps the strength of the others in the household; this may be the factor that tips the balance against remaining at home.

Abrupt change in status relatively early in the terminal illness sometimes requires hospitalization for evaluation. A patient who is otherwise doing very well and suddenly develops weakness and paresthesia in the legs may require more careful assessment than can be provided at home.

Sometimes a brief period of hospitalization is provided largely to give rest to an exhausted or sick caregiver at home. Admission to the hospital for this purpose may raise questions about reimbursement for inpatient care from third party payors. It points up the need for a hospital-based program with home care to have available an intermediate care facility in which hospice care can be provided without loss of continuity. Our program and most hospital-based programs do not have such an arrangement. However, the issue seldom presents a practical problem. In most cases in which the primary purpose of hospitalization is to provide respite for a caregiver at home, the need occurs because of specific physical problems which the patient has; these can legitimately be cited as the reasons for hospitalization. One must concede that this is a grey area, but the author has no personal difficulty in justifying hospitalization in these circumstances because, over the long haul, hospice care is cost effective; this is simply one of the built-in costs. In other words, without hospice care such a patient would probably have spent a much larger share of his terminal illness in the hospital under more costly circumstances.

Each patient and his family are dealt with on an individual basis to determine in what setting optimal care can be rendered. Ready access to and smooth transition between various levels of care are essential to optimal management of the terminally ill, as are excellent communication and co-ordination between personnel providing care at those levels.

Using all that morphine, aren't patients knocked out and don't they get addicted?

Addiction is not a problem in the terminally ill. To begin with, the course of most patients is of such a nature that addiction is irrelevant. Furthermore, our experience, and that of others, has been that patients with chronic pain from advanced malignancy are able to reduce the dosage of narcotic without serious problem if, for some reason, pain is relieved by other means, such as radiation therapy.

An observation that has been made repeatedly with respect to the use of drugs for the relief of chronic pain in terminal illness is that for most narcotics there is a range of dosage within which the patient can be maintained free of pain and quite alert. The only drowsiness that most patients experience is during the initial period of dosage adjustment when they are being brought into that range.

In patients for whom severe pain has been a problem for a time, we begin by assuring the patient at the outset that we can relieve his pain without rendering him somnolent. We start with a quite heavy dosage of narcotic, which may produce drowsiness. We then gradually back off into that range of dosage that leaves him quite bright but pain free. From time to time, advancing disease will result in increased pain, in which instance narcotic dosage can usually be increased to satisfactory analgesic levels without producing drowsiness. One really has to see hospice patients alert and comfortable on what we would ordinarily consider prohibitive doses of morphine to truly comprehend how well this works.

Aside from those in the process of initial dosage adjustment, the only drowsy, indolent patients are those who are extremely debilitated. Most of these patients are at a stage in their terminal illness at which they would exhibit lassitude even without narcotic administration. Debility does, however, seem to narrow that range of narcotic dosage within which the patient can be maintained pain free and alert.

Do you permit connubial visits?

Yes. In our program, however, this has rarely been a consideration because most patients who are well enough to be sexually active are not on the inpatient unit. In those few exceptions our hospice staff has discretely demonstrated its imagination, ingenuity and compassion in arranging connubial visits.

Do you let patients take drugs like Laetrile?

We discourage the use of measures such as Laetrile on two grounds. First, such substances appear to be medically useless and sometimes harmful. Second, condoning the use of what the patient sees as curative therapy runs counter to the type of adjustment that we are usually hoping the patient will make to his situation.

As a practical matter, there is no way in which we can prevent a patient from popping an occasional Laetrile. However, this is usually not the fashion in which the drug is administered by its advocates. It is given as part of a program which includes special diets, megavitamins and high colonic irrigations. We have found these measures to be quite incompatible with hospice care.

Laetrile is only the unapproved form of cancer treatment currently most highly publicized. There are many other similar programs available at various places throughout the world. Our attitude toward all of these is the same as our attitude toward Laetrile.

Do you experiment on hospice patients?

Hospice patients are not used as the subjects of clinical studies of anti-tumor therapy. Even for symptomatic treatment, previously untested treatment schemes are not employed. However, we do try to learn as much as we can from our experience with each patient.

Why do patients drop out of the program?

Once entered, very few patients drop out of the hospice program. Because of the particular course of their disease, some patients require little or no hospice service over a protracted period of time. Such patients are at home and regular home care visits would be superfluous. Because many home care services are not reimbursed by third party payors, the patient and his family may request cessation of home care services because of concern about expense. Such patients are maintained on inactive status. Contact with them is not lost and they are returned to active status as soon as hospice care services are deemed warranted.

There are several reasons why a very small number of patients (less than 2%) have left the program before death. In spite of admission screening, which attempts to assure that the patient's home situation makes home care possible, the home situation may be misjudged or may change for some reason, such as the illness or death of a family member. In such cases, it may be necessary to place the patient in a nursing home where all aspects of hospice care can not be provided. Our program presently is capable of providing inhospital care and care at home, but we have no formal mechanism for continuing hospice care in an intermediate facility such as a nursing home. Negotiations are presently under way to fill this gap.

There are a few other reasons for withdrawal from the program. Error in diagnosis at the time of admission can occur. The importance of avoiding this if possible and of recognizing it promptly if it does occur is obvious. Although we have seen a number of instances of partial spontaneous remission of tumor in our hospice patients, we have not yet had an instance of complete and permanent spontaneous regression. Such a patient would probably be put on inactive status rather than dropped from the program. The same applies to unanticipated therapeutic remissions.

Two patients have been withdrawn from the program by their attending physicians. In one case this was for the purpose of instituting vigorous anti-tumor therapy, presumably in the hope of cure. In the other instance the attending physician wished, very late in the patient's course, to provide vigorous supportive treatment in the form of intravenous solutions and endotracheal intubation; such aggressive treatment is simply incompatible with principles of hospice care.

After a patient has been entered into the program he, or sometimes the family, may have a change of heart about accepting inevitability of incurability and may decide to abandon the program to undertake anti-tumor therapy. Sometimes they do this through conventional avenues such as radiation or chemotherapy, but usually it has been to participate in unapproved treatments such as the use of Laetrile. A few patients leave a hospice program simply because they feel that they can handle the situation on their own.

Although we are naturally disheartened whenever a patient is withdrawn from the program, we have learned a great deal from these experiences. The matter of withdrawal by the attending physician deserves some special comment. It is in a sense part of the price we pay for allowing referring physicians on our staff the option of continuing as the patient's attending physician in the hospice care program. It has been a small price for a valuable feature of the program and is a problem that can probably be corrected with additional physician education.

However, as can be seen from the two instances in which this occurred, the problem goes beyond the hospice care program. The patients cited at least entered the program. The real problem is to identify how frequently such decisions are made *before* entry into a hospice program, so that patients who might profit are kept out of the program. This is a matter that requires the attention of all physicians concerned with improving the care of the terminally ill. We are attempting to study this subject through our departmental audit committees and our quality assurance program.

What about the special problems of the dying child?

Church Hospital has Medical, Surgical and Gynecological services. It does not have a Pediatric service and does not admit children below the adolescent level. Therefore, we have not taken children into our hospice care program.

Many of the problems and principles of caring for the dying adult apply also to the dying child; there are naturally some special considerations in children. Some hospice programs have had experience with children, but for the most part this has been quite limited.

In part, this is because deaths from malignant disease are relatively uncommon in children and adolescents. This means that it is unlikely for any one hospice program to gain a wide experience with children.

The work of Martinson (1980) indicates that the establishment of carefully developed home care programs offers the most promising approach in dealing with terminally ill children and adolescents and their families. Increased knowledge about the handling of death and dying and increased development of programs that utilize available existing knowledge are among the major needs in the years ahead.

References

Breindel, C.L. and Gravely, G.E.: *Costs of Providing a Mixed-Unit Hospice Program.* Working paper, Dept. Health Administration, Medical College of Virginia (1980)

Martinson, I.M.: *Dying Children at Home.*

International Hospice Conference (1980)

Twycross, R.G.: Clinical experience with diamorphine in advanced malignant disease. Intern J Clin Pharmacol Ther Toxicol, Vol. 9, 184 (1974)

10. The Future of Hospice Care

Hospice care for the terminally ill has reached the point where it is time to take stock of where we have been and where we are. But if we are to meet our full potential, we must also look ahead to where we are going. As we look ahead there are two questions we should ask. What is the future likely to do to us? What can we do to the future? The answer to neither question carries any degree of certainty but, troubling as uncertainty is, we must not allow it to paralyze progress.

The focus of what follows is not upon where we are being taken, but upon where we need to go. Nonetheless, it is important to examine the forces that are likely to shape our options.

Uncertain economic and international conditions notwithstanding, it is difficult to foresee circumstances under which there will not be continuing growth of hospice care programs. An increasing interest in and willingness to confront the handling of death and terminal illness, coupled with the results of hospice care programs in action, constitute a compelling argument for the wider use of such programs. Most indications seem to point the way toward expansion of hospice care. The experience of our program and that of others indicates that in most communities there is a need for additional hospice programs.

One of the strengths of hospice thus far has been its diversity of form and style (Osterweis and Champagne, 1979). Successful hospice programs have adapted to local needs. We hope this will continue. Some free-standing hospices have obviously been enormously productive and have provided valuable knowledge regarding the care of the terminally ill. In some circumstances they will be the best means of meeting community needs. However, the Church Hospital hospice experience and that of other hospital-affiliated programs confirm that the hospital-based hospice is not only a possible but also a desirable alternative approach.

There are philosophic, organizational and financial reasons for promoting the growth of hospital-based units. We hope to see the development and expansion of various types of hospital-based programs. Some will possess a separate facility for hospice patients; some, like Church Hospital's, will have hospice patients integrated with non-hospice patients on a nursing unit; some will have hospice patients distributed throughout the hospital under treatment by a palliative care team. As new programs are contemplated, those responsible for starting them should examine the options carefully and should design the programs best suited to their particular circumstances. Standards for hospice care must be drawn so as to permit this diversity.

As time passes it would perhaps be well if the distinctions between free-standing and hospital-based hospices are blurred. Possibly each hospice program will continue to have a locus at which its administrative function is centered. This may be in a hospital, in a free-standing unit or in a home care program. However, hospitals, free-standing units and home care programs serve patients at different levels of care. What is most needed for optimal care of the terminally ill are programs that are truly comprehensive in that they offer continuity of care as the patient shifts from one level to another. In other words, hospice programs should be organized so as to enable the application of hospice principles and practice across the entire spectrum.

It will be imperative for hospital-based programs to offer care not only in the hospital but in the home, as well as to patients who require institutionalization in an intermediate care facility. For many the term nursing home carries very unpleasant connotations. However, there is nothing that makes it categorically impossible for the finest type of hospice care to be available within a nursing home setting. Just as there is nothing which mandates that a hospital providing acute general care cannot offer excellent hospice care, so there is nothing which dictates that a nursing home facility providing care to other patients cannot also render hospice care of the highest caliber. Hospital-based hospice programs should seek to develop suitable arrangements so that they can provide care at the intermediate and home care levels. Often this will require arrangements with existing intermediate care facilities.

Similarly, free-standing hospice units will need to develop formalized arrangements that will permit the preservation of continuity of care when patients require acute hospital care. They will also have to cultivate the types of relationships that permit easy transition between levels of care. They must be certain that patients who would profit from some of the techniques that hospitalization allows are not denied the advantages which this would permit.

Programs that begin with a home care base will need to find the means whereby patients can receive care in intermediate facilities and in hospitals without loss of continuity of care.

In other words, whatever the origin and whatever the center of operations, the ultimate aim of hospice programs is going to have to be the provision of comprehensive care. Otherwise, hospice will run the danger of perpetuating the kind of fragmentation which has plagued the conventional approach which it seeks to replace.

Clarification of cost and reimbursement issues must be concomitant with resolution of the organizational problems in hospice care. Decisions in these areas are matters of public policy and will have to be addressed in this fashion. The health consumer will have to determine for what he wishes to pay. The role of hospice leaders in this is to inform the public of what is available, so that consumers can make intelligent choices.

There are a number of questions to be dealt with. Is care of the terminally ill important, or should our financial resources be directed primarily at curative and rehabilitative medicine? If we are to reimburse for terminal care, what services should be reimbursed? Should bereavement counseling be reimbursable? At what level should services be reimbursed? What sort of organizational format should we require of those providing terminal care in order to be eligible for reimbursement? Should only hospital-based programs or only free-standing programs be eligible? What stipulations and restrictions should be placed upon the delivery of care at home? Should it be necessary that the patient be homebound?

It is the legislatures and insurance companies, presumably on the basis of public preference, which establish the services that will be reimbursed and the formulae for that reimbursement. They need to be particularly well informed about issues relating to the care of the terminally ill.

Through the experience of free-standing and hospital-based programs and of third party payors such as Blue Cross, some data are now being gathered with respect to costs and reimbursement problems in hospice care. Certain demonstration projects (for example, that sponsored by the Health Care Financing Administration) are experimenting with waivers on some of the restrictions on reimbursement for home care, such as the homebound requirement. However, it is debatable whether such experiments will provide us with definitive answers for the future. This type of study, done on a limited basis for a small, identifiable and carefully selected group of programs, may not yield information which can be transferred to a more universal situation. Nonetheless, it is a beginning.

The resolution of cost and reimbursement issues may result in other problems. In its formative years, hospice care has been characterized by a high level of altruism among its personnel. As hospice services become reimbursable, the potential for exploitation is inevitable. This is going to require the vigilance of conscientious hospice leaders.

As hospice systems evolve and matters of reimbursement are settled, the role of volunteers in hospice care will require close scrutiny and careful thought. The contribution of volunteers to the success of hospice has been enormous. This contribution has in part been through the provision of services which have made the volunteers effective extenders of the professionals on the health care team. This has had a tremendous financial impact. In some instances, it has made hospice care possible, for it is only in this way that the high level of personal attention which hospice care requires could be provided. But, in addition, volunteers have contributed in another important respect; they have brought values and viewpoints that have refreshed and strengthened hospice programs.

To the extent that hospice care becomes more integrated into the health care system, as accreditation of hospice programs develops and as reimbursement for hospice care becomes more widely available, there is clearly a threat to volunteer involvement in hospice. The necessary steps must be taken to preserve volunteer participation.

Among those of us who have looked carefully at hospice care, one of the principal concerns has been the relationship between hospice care in particular and medical care in general. There are innumerable forms which this relationship could take. At one extreme is the frightening prospect of a totally separate system for the care of the terminally ill, entirely outside of and completely unrelated to the rest of health care. Serious hospice workers would be less than realistic if they considered unthinkable the development of a cult-like phenomenon for the care of the terminally ill. At the opposite extreme is the thought that within the hospice concept are the seeds of a healthy self-destruction, in the course of which hospice care would become completely amalgamated into general medical care perfusing many of its precepts into the management of acutely ill patients. In truth, it is improbable that the future will take us to either of these extremes. As is often the case, the central part of the spectrum seems not only more sensible, but also more likely.

A number of features of the care of the terminally ill suggest that management of such patients will in some respects be a specialty, but one comfortably within the framework of the traditional medical care system. The unique problems faced by the dying are of such a nature as to merit the special attention of certain physicians. There will always be a sizable number of physicians who, confronted with patients who reach the stage of terminal disease, do not, for one reason or another, wish to be responsible for the continuing care of the patient. Surgeons, radiotherapists and oncologists are particularly likely to fall in this group. Their reasons for not wishing to continue in the care of the patient are usually sound and we would be prudent to honor them.

Thus the need to provide terminal care and the need to find means to improve that terminal care will direct us toward the development of a specialty in the care of the terminally ill. This specialty will be particularly fortunate to be able to look with pride at founders of unusual depth, compassion and character. Cicely Saunders, Tom West, Eric Wilkes, Richard Lamerton, Balfour Mount, Sylvia Lack, Bill Lamers and others are providing a legacy that should be the foundation of an honorable history.

Specialties come in all degrees. Whether care of the terminally ill will become so discrete and well developed as to have its own certifying board depends upon a number of imponderables. Whatever direction it takes, it is clear that hospice care will have a major impact upon this specialty. Hospice care is not likely to evaporate, leaving no trace of itself. In this connection we must remember that care of the terminally ill and hospice care as we know it today are not synonymous.

Entirely outside of and completely unrelated to hospice care there seem to be some healthy changes taking place in dealing with malignant disease and terminally ill patients. For example, in the surgical literature there has been a subtle but definite shift in emphasis with respect to the treatment of patients with lesions such as esophageal carcinoma. A few years ago, results of treatment were reported in terms of cure rates, usually winding up with an overall figure in the range of a 5 to 10% 5-year survival rate. Nothing was said about the 90 to 95% of patients who were not cured. Recently, there has been an increasing recognition that our present modes of treatment for esophageal carcinoma are best looked at in terms of the palliation they provide, with cure being achieved in a minority of patients. This in no way denies the importance of a continuing search for techniques that will result in cure.

It is the author's impression that we do not often see a senseless prolongation of life without reason or meaning, even outside of hospice care. Such cases do occur, but they are relatively rare. It has been the author's experience that the situation has usually arisen because there was at one point in the patient's course a time when resuscitation and rehabilitation seemed advisable; once having begun the use of life support systems, it is very difficult to discontinue them.

In November 1978, the Board of Trustees and House of Delegates of the American Medical Association passed a resolution pledging to actively encourage and implement continued education of the practicing physician in the most effective methods "for meeting the symptomatic, rehabilitative, supportive and other needs of the cancer patient." In conformity with this resolution, the Journal of the American Medical Association has initiated a series of articles on care of the patient with advanced cancer (Moertel, 1980).

The point is that in the management of the terminally ill there are healthy changes taking place entirely apart from hospice care. To some extent these are a product of the same forces that have given birth to and shaped hospice programs.

If care of the terminally ill is to develop as some form of specialty, hospice care is likely to be a part of it. Hospice care possess some features which make it different from any other medical specialty. One of these is the liberal use of many disciplines and of volunteers. Non-medical people have played an immense role in the development and conduct of hospice care. They bring to those of us in medicine some perspectives and insights which we would not otherwise have. It is to be hoped that they will continue to give of themselves so generously and that the response of physicians and other medical people will be positive. We must watch for and avoid two dangers. Non-medical people interested in seeing hospice care develop may become so strident that they discourage the participation of medical people and then so frustrated that they decide to move outside the existing health care system. Conversely, medical people may become defensive about what they see as criticism of the way in which they are doing things; they may cease to listen.

The matters of standards and certification deserve and unquestionably will receive considerable attention in the years ahead. Care of the terminally ill and hospice care are not alone in this. However, because they are relatively young as identifiable areas for attention and because they possess certain features that are particularly prone to abuse, they will have to deal with some special issues. Problems related to the lack of restriction on the use of the term hospice also raise some unusual questions.

The National Hospice Organization has taken the initiative in developing standards for hospices. This is a most important matter and should be pursued vigorously. Several considerations must be borne in mind as standards for hospice care are formulated. As in all areas of medical care, standards must not become an impediment to progress, stamping everyone into a mold of mediocrity. It is particularly important in hospice care that there be enough flexibility to permit diversity and innovation. It is equally important that the initiative for setting and enforcing standards remain with those in the field of hospice care, rather than in the hands of government agencies.

Even within this framework an issue that will have to be faced for hospital-based hospices is the relationship between the National Hospice Organization and the Joint Commission on Accreditation of Hospitals. It is hoped that suitable arrangements can be made to prevent overlapping and conflicting requirements or the need for two separate certifications. Actually cooperation between the two agencies can strengthen the accreditation process as it relates to the care of the terminally ill.

In addition to certification or accreditation of hospices, there is the issue of assessing the quality of care within hospices. The Joint Commission on Accreditation of Hospitals requires that all hospitals have a mechanism for assuring quality of care. It is important that each hospital that treats terminally ill patients apply these mechanisms to the evaluation of care of those patients whether or not it has a hospice care program. Quality assurance through audit can be a demanding and time consuming process, but hospital-affiliated hospice programs should be certain that they are included in the medical care evaluation process in the hospital. This requires the setting of criteria and the review of data.

Hospice care is clearly maturing. Whether it is in its infancy, childhood or adolescence is not entirely clear. What is clear is that it still has some growing up to do. It must begin to learn to face the responsibilities of adulthood.

Like all of medical care, hospice care contains a large measure of *art*. Artistic skill requires development through discipline and learning. There is still much progress to be made in the art of hospice care; what follows is in no way intended to de-emphasize this aspect of the care of the terminally ill.

What must receive careful attention from hospice workers in the future, however, is the care of the terminally ill as a developing *science*. The groundwork in most scientific fields has been descriptive. However, to grow and flourish and make a contribution to humanity, a science must go beyond this. Hospice care is ready to do this and needs to do it. Up to this point, much of hospice care has been defined in anecdotal terms. It is now time to begin to gather and analyze data by the scientific method and to test hypotheses.

This raises in many minds, most particularly in those of non-medical people interested in hospice care, the issue of experimentation. All of us in hospice care must learn not to be ashamed of the word "research." Only through research can we reach full fruition. There is no reason why the terms research and experimentation should connote for the hospice worker images of cruel and grueling treatment, for research can be conducted with the utmost human compassion. Research in the care of the terminally ill will be demanding, but it will be demanding of the researchers, not of the patients.

An early step which will be a particularly challenging one will involve the development of measurement tools. This will at times seem to defy efforts. The objective of hospice care is the control of symptoms in the broadest sense of that term. Symptoms, whether physical or psychological, are by their nature subjective. Measurement of subjective phenomena is difficult, but not impossible. Hospice workers, who have the advantage of already being geared to a multidisciplinary approach, must be ready to draw upon a variety of fields in which subjective factors are measured. Techniques applicable to hospice patients have doubtless already been developed; the time has come for their application. The capacity to assess the degree of relief of pain, weakness, nausea, anxiety and depression will open important vistas for hospice care.

As in all scientific endeavor, the adequacy of measurement tools is the subject of endless debate. This is particularly true of measurement tools used to assess subjective phenomena. We must indeed preserve our skepticism and continue to question the methods we employ; that is part of science. However, we must not allow that debate to stop all progress. We can not allow ourselves to say that because we cannot measure something precisely, we should not measure it at all.

Measurement tools that relate not to symptom relief but to the organization and cost of hospice care, need to be developed. Some new techniques for quantification of personnel time and program component costs should be developed. Many of these techniques already exist and only need to be applied, perhaps with some modification.

As measurement tools are developed they can and should be applied by hospice workers to study a number of problems. There clearly needs to be comparison of hospice care with other forms of care for the terminally ill. Up to this point, our efforts to promote the development of hospice care have been hinged largely to our descriptions and anecdotes. Those we are trying to convince will soon rightfully be demanding more from us. They will want some data; we should be ready to provide them. It is only in this way that growth of hospice care can be unfettered.

There is even greater need, however, for the application of research techniques within hospice care; there is a need for the comparison of various techniques of hospice care. Although we have done better with some symptoms than others, we have not yet reached perfection in handling any. We must apply acceptable measurement tools to the study of alternative methods of treatment of symptoms. It is when this is done that we can begin to reap the full fruits of what hospice care has to offer.

We also need to apply our measurement tools to the relative merits of different organizational structures within hospice care. It is through such study that we can begin to make more rational decisions regarding the selection of a model of hospice care for a given community.

An area to which some investigative effort should be directed is the question of the effect of hospice care on the *quantity* of life. Since the overall goal of a program for the care of the terminally ill is the expansion of both the quantity and quality of life, the impact of various treatment measures on duration of survival can be useful information in making clinical decisions. The effect of various forms of therapy on survival duration has, of course, a financial as well as clinical dimension; knowledge about this can be helpful.

Some other areas of investigation relating to the care of the terminally ill suggest themselves. For example, we know little today about the mechanisms by which malignant disease produces symptoms or even about the mechanism of death from advanced malignancy. Some of us believe that there is reason to question the widely accepted view that pneumonia is the final common pathway of death in most patients with advanced cancer.

Some beginnings have been made in the application of the scientific method to the care of the terminally ill in general and to hospice care in particular. Recognizing that in no field will science solve all of our problems by giving us definitive answers to our most important questions, we must move ahead in our effort to answer as many questions as possible.

Just as hospice care must be, fundamentally, a medical program in order to reach its full potential, it must also have its roots firmly in science. We are in an era when there has indeed been a "flight from science" (Editorial, 1980). Historically, methods of alternative medicine have made some of their heaviest inroads in the area of care of the terminally ill. Hospice care owes much of its success to basic and clinical science and will do well to keep its attachments to them.

Conversely, this is also an era in which increasingly prevalent regulatory mechanisms have emphasized an extremely technological and disease-oriented approach to the treatment of patients. Our reimbursement systems are increasingly ignoring the contribution of personal attention to medical care (Burnum, 1979). This development bears watching by hospice workers in the years ahead.

One interesting and anomalous feature of hospice care is that, in England and in the United States, it has developed so largely outside our academic institutions. This is surprising because it has been so seldom in the last several decades that medicine has seen something as valuable and with as much potential impact as hospice care develop with so little input from major medical centers and universities. Notwithstanding the closer relationship of Canadian hospices or palliative care programs to medical schools and recognizing the role of a few institutions such as Georgetown University, the lack of involvement on the part of American teaching centers has been striking.

It is interesting to speculate upon possible reasons for this. Understanding these reasons may contribute to correcting what can only be seen as an unfortunate situation. Nonetheless, the only point to be made here is the desirability of university involvement in hospice care in the future. Some might say that if we have gotten this far without them, we do not need them now; they may just complicate things. For several reasons, we do need their interest, support and involvement. University medical centers are the repositories of resources which hospices need. They possess educational capabilities; it is through the introduction of medical students and house officers to hospice care as a part of the fabric of medical practice that we can hope to see the widespread application of hospice principles to the terminally ill. University medical centers have the research capacity, expertise and experience which can be so valuable to the future care of the terminally ill. This is not to suggest that every university hospital needs to open a hospice care unit. There are various means by which academic centers can become involved in hospice care; such involvement would be to the advantage of both the universities and hospices. Put another way, academic institutions and major medical centers possess talents and a stature in our society which can only be ignored at some peril.

On the basis of experience thus far it would appear that the approach embodied in the philosophy and practice of hospice care offers the potential for improved care of the terminally ill at a reasonable cost. Hospice programs are likely to increase in numbers and sophistication. Both the art and science of hospice care will grow as experience is gained. Hospice care can reach its full potential as it becomes an integral part of our medical care system. The needs of dying patients and their loved ones demand no less.

References

Burnum, J.R.: Scientific Value of Personal Care. Ann Intern Med, Vol. 91, 643 (1979)

Editorial. The Flight from Science. Br Med J, Vol. 280, 1 (1980)

Moertel, C.G.: Care of the Patient with Advanced Cancer. JAMA, Vol. 244, 175 (1980)

Osterweis, M.; Champagne, D.S.: The U.S. Hospice Movement; Issues in Development. Am J Public Health, Vol. 69, 492 (1979)

Index

185